THE "ACCI"

THE "ACCI"

How the Birmingham Accident Hospital led the World in the management of the severely injured

IAN GREAVES

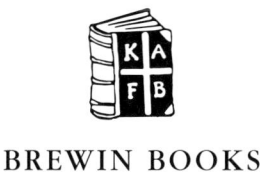

BREWIN BOOKS

BREWIN BOOKS
19 Enfield Ind. Estate,
Redditch,
Worcestershire,
B97 6BY
www.brewinbooks.com

Published by Brewin Books 2023

© Ian Greaves, 2023

The author has asserted his rights in accordance with the Copyright, Designs and Patents Act 1988 to be identified as the author of this work.

All rights reserved. No part of this publication may be reproduced, stored in a retrieval system, or transmitted in any form or by any means, electronic, mechanical, photocopying, recording or otherwise, without the prior permission in writing of the publisher and the copyright owners, or as expressly permitted by law, or under terms agreed with the appropriate reprographics rights organisation. Enquiries concerning reproduction outside the terms stated here should be sent to the publishers at the UK address printed on this page.

The publisher makes no representation, express or implied, with regard to the accuracy of the information contained in this book and cannot accept any legal responsibility for any errors or omissions that may be made.

A CIP catalogue record for this book is available from the British Library.

ISBN: 978-1-85858-762-2 (Paperback)
ISBN: 978-1-85858-763-9 (Hardback)

Printed and bound in Great Britain
by Bell & Bain Ltd.

Contents

Foreword	ix
Preface	x
Acknowledgements and Picture Credits	xi
Introduction – The Fourth Horseman	xiii
Prelude – Temple Row, Birmingham 1825	xviii
1. Foundations	1
2. A Hospital at War	14
First Interlude – The Birth of Orthopaedics	34
3. A Hospital at Work and at Play	43
4. State of the Art	53
Second Interlude – Why do Trauma Patients Die?	68
5. Surgery on Wheels and in the Air	75
Third Interlude – 21st November 1974	82
6. Still Innovating	87
7. The Head Injuries Club	94
Fourth Interlude – War and Peace	102
8. Closure	107
9. A Hospital at War Again	112
Afterword	118
Further Reading	121
Index	122

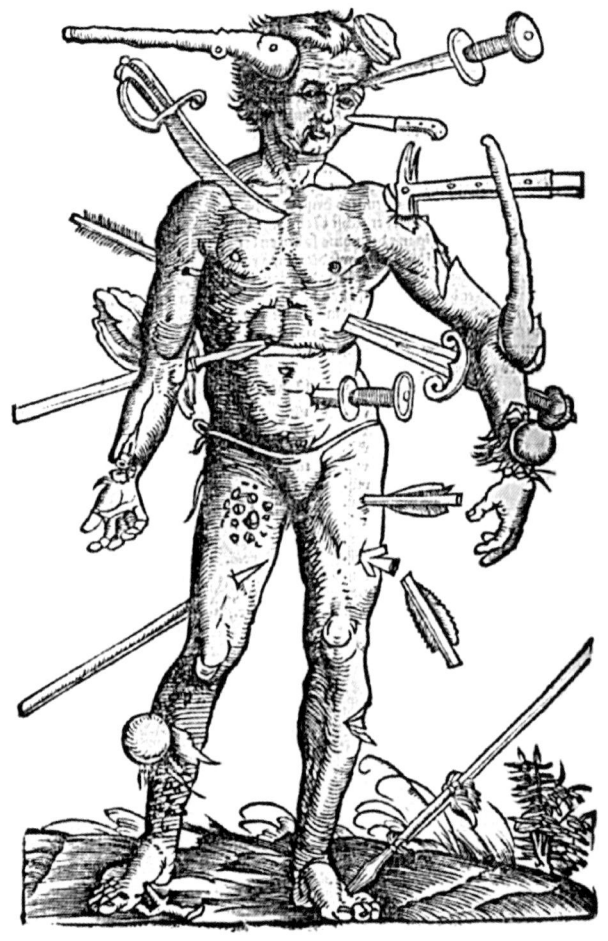

The "wound man" from Hans von Gersdorff's Feldtbuch der Wundartzney *printed in Strasburg in the early sixteenth century.*

This book is dedicated to my late parents Bob and Margaret Greaves without whose love, sacrifices and commitment I would never have got to Birmingham in the first place and to all those who once worked at their beloved "Acci".

* * *

The author's royalties from this book have been donated to support the work of the educational and research charity TRAUMA CARE.

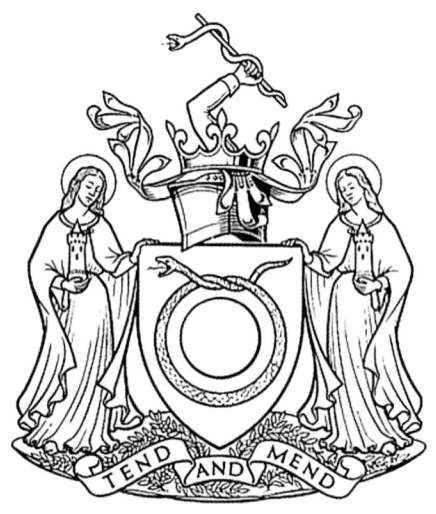

The coat of Arms of the Institute of Accident Surgery at the Birmingham Accident Hospital.

Foreword by Professor Sir Keith Porter Kt CStJ FRCS

Formerly consultant trauma surgeon, Birmingham Accident Hospital. Retired consultant surgeon, Queen Elizabeth Hospital and Royal Centre for Defence Medicine. Formerly Professor of Clinical Traumatology, University of Birmingham.

AS ALDOUS HUXLEY remarked, *"That men do not learn much from the lessons of History is the most important of all the lessons that history has to teach."* Sadly, medicine provides many examples of the truth of this aphorism and there is no more striking example than that of the Birmingham Accident Hospital (*The Acci*). It would be more than 20 years after the closure of the Accident Hospital before major trauma centres embracing many of the principles and practices developed and founded at *The Acci* were established in England.

It is therefore vital that the history of *The Acci*, its people and the services it provided are captured as a record of the legacy of those who dedicated their lives to the care of the injured there and in doing so created the World's first dedicated trauma hospital.

This book captures not only the history of the hospital but the development of trauma services in general. It makes reference to the teamwork and camaraderie amongst the staff of the Birmingham Accident Hospital and also to many of its ground-breaking achievements, including understanding shock and blood resuscitation, burn management, trauma critical care and care of the trauma victim "in the round" from injury to rehabilitation. Also revealed is the hospital's global reputation through its research departments for its work on wound microbiology, infection control and accident prevention. Modern clinicians will find striking contrasts between hospital life then and now.

Many of the principles of treatment which were developed at *The Acci* later formed the basis of military medical practice and in turn evolved over time to guide the care delivered in the theatres of war in Afghanistan and Iraq, as well as at the Centre for Defence Medicine at Birmingham's Queen Elizabeth Hospital.

As the last trauma surgeon appointed to the hospital, I felt it was essential to capture and share so many memories from this wonderful institution which was revered by medical staff the world over and much loved by the people of the West Midlands that it served so loyally; hence my commission to the author, Professor Ian Greaves, a distinguished medical author and himself an Accident Hospital alumnus. All royalties from the book will be donated to the charity *Trauma Care*. I very much hope you will enjoy it.

Preface

WHEN I WAS a medical student at Birmingham University Medical School in the first half of the 1980s, the Birmingham Accident Hospital, known to everyone as *The Acci* had achieved near mythical status. It was where many of us, at an early point in our training – which would surprise today's students, gained our first experience of stitching and other simple procedures, we knew that *The Acci* was something special. The United Kingdom does not have a glorious history of managing the victims of trauma; indeed it was only after a series of critical reports repeatedly highlighted inadequacies in such care, that today's system of trauma centres and trauma networks was finally established in the second decade of the twenty-first century. And yet, from its foundation in 1941, the Birmingham Accident Hospital, formerly the Queen's Hospital Birmingham, was a centre of excellence in the treatment of the victims of trauma.

Those of us who were lucky enough to work at *The Acci* remember its very special atmosphere and look back with sadness at its demise. I suspect every doctor remembers his first time "on the wards". Mine was at the Birmingham Accident Hospital and I remember fondly sitting at a long table in the middle of a long ward lit only by a single lamp. In addition, its surviving veterans are becoming increasingly thin on the ground and memories fade with age. But there is no doubt that small hospitals, now few in number, generated loyalty in a way few if any of today's huge centres do. In reality, however, the tradition of first-rate trauma care simply moved, first to the General Hospital, then to Selly Oak Hospital and finally to the Queen Elizabeth Hospital, where the foundations were laid for the trauma service which served the injured personnel from the wars in Iraq and Afghanistan so well and continues to serve the people of the West Midlands.

The story of the Birmingham Accident Hospital began in 1825. By the time it closed in 1993, its clinicians had included pioneers of surgery, anaesthesia, radiology and the treatment of burns, but above all doctors, nurses, radiographers, physiotherapists and a whole host of others from porters to secretaries who all believed in *The Acci,* were proud to be a part of it and worked as a team to offer integrated care of the highest possible quality to the victims of trauma. Where *The Acci* led, others, sooner or later, would follow.

It is all too easy to believe that the World's first major trauma centre was in Baltimore, New York or Boston, or possibly even in Johannesburg or London, but it wasn't; it was in Birmingham, it was The Birmingham Accident Hospital and this is its story.

Acknowledgements

IT IS CONVENTIONAL for the author's acknowledgements to appear at the end of a book, but they appear here because without the work of the following people, this book would never have been written and the history of the Birmingham Accident Hospital (BAH) and its contribution to modern medicine might have been left in increasing obscurity. It is with thanks and great pleasure, therefore, that I recognise the contributions of the following who have shared their reminiscences of working at the BAH: Professor Howard Champion, Dr Graeme Dickson, Mr John Gower, Maggie Horner and Dr Anne Sutcliffe. Peter Millard kindly provided details of the hospital's Royal visits. My friend from the year of 1986, Dr John Etherington CBE, kindly shared his expertise and experience of clinical rehabilitation services in the UK. Roger Farrell and Michael Walker kindly offered their memories of the Birmingham Pub Bombings. My friend of 30 years, Professor Sir Keith Porter, was always available as a source of information and advice: thank you. I would also like to thank my wife Julia for putting up with yet another project.

My principle and greatest debt, however, is to Hatty Tovey who so diligently carried out the original research in the Birmingham Accident Hospital archives and undertook the interviews with former BAH employees. This book simply would not have been written without her.

Picture Credits
The image of Dr John Bull on page 65 is a Central Office of Information photograph: Crown Copyright Reserved. The majority of the images are taken from The Birmingham Accident Hospital archives or are in the public domain.

Αἰέν ἀριστεύέιν

....

*"This hospital does not treat accidents
but the people suffering from accidents."*

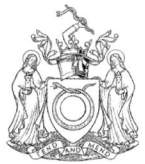

Introduction

The Fourth Horseman

OTHER PEOPLE'S INJURIES, whether fictional or real, appear, along with interior decoration, gardening and cooking, to have become a national obsession. From the travails of the staff of Holby City's crisis ridden emergency department in BBC One's *Casualty* to the endless fly-on-the-wall documentaries, there seems to be a general fascination with other people's trauma. Helicopters and doctors in orange suits appear to be a particularly potent combination in the public imagination, a combination of *deus ex machina* and shameless self-promotion.

There has also been a thread of trauma through medical culture and especially medical comedy, focusing on small boys with pans on their heads (something that almost never happens in real life) and foreign bodies in places one would not expect to find them. The latter is a favourite area for competitive dinner party comparison amongst doctors, the tally amongst my own patients includes a bust of Napoleon, a walking stick (bent end), a crown cork remover, vegetables (assorted), low calorie olive oil spray, the inevitable vibrator and several small furry animals; all recently topped by a World War II shell requiring bomb disposal as well as clinical intervention.

All this having been said, the public has never really engaged with trauma in the same way that it has thrown itself behind cancer care, HIV or even COVID. There has never been, and perhaps never will be, a demand from the public to ensure that the victims of trauma receive the best possible care. Unfortunately, this lack of demand for coordinated action was mirrored amongst the medical profession until very recently. If it might be said that the three horsemen of the modern medical apocalypse (updating the traditional Death, Famine, War, and Conquest) are Starvation, Infection and Climate Change; then the fourth is Trauma. It has been estimated that between 14,000 and 16,000 people Worldwide die each day as a result of trauma: five million annual deaths each year or almost 10% of Worldwide deaths. Trauma is the cause of death in 25% of those who die between the ages of 15 and 44 but it is believed that the mortality might be even higher in the elderly. So-called "silver trauma", serious or life-threatening injury following what initially appears to be a trivial accident, is now increasingly recognised as a cause of mortality amongst older people.

If the number of deaths due to trauma is a matter of concern, the number of lives blighted is even more alarming. Although the effects of trauma on those who do not die are difficult to measure, social scientists have developed the concept of *disability-adjusted life years (DALYs)*, as a measure of years lived with disability following trauma: one DALY is one lost year of healthy life. It has been suggested that injuries are responsible for 15% of Worldwide DALYs. Given the scale of the trauma pandemic, and that presumably trauma has been common since ancient man stuck a spear in his foot or got a flint chip in his eye, it would seem obvious that the medical profession has devoted centuries of effort to finding and refining the treatment of the injured. Obvious, but wrong. In practice, doctors have traditionally been rather sniffy about the injured, leaving the management of fractures to unqualified bone setters, or, and historically almost as bad, to those members of the profession who served with the fighting men and later the armed forces of their nations.

There is evidence from earlier times in the archaeological remains of patients who survived broken bones and infections arising from injuries. Some individuals show signs of being trepanned, a process in which a part of the skull is removed. This is now recognised as a treatment for raised pressure within the skull following trauma, which is designed to protect the brain from damage. Although it was probably first used as a means of releasing evil spirits from those possessed, it does appear to have been used in ancient times in those who had suffered head injury. It is clear that a method of stabilising fractures whilst they healed was also available from earlier times, presumably this consisted of pieces of wood fastened to the limb with some kind of tie. As we shall see, plaster of Paris is a very recent addition to fracture treatment but after the battles of the Crusades, bandages soaked in horses' blood did provide some degree of effective splintage as the blood dried. There was at least some logic behind this remedy as there is behind using honey as a wound dressing or maggots to remove dead tissue, both practices current in the Middle Ages. An alternative Crusader treatment for fractures (and also for hernias) was *mummia*, a powder of ground up Egyptian mummies. Both *mummia* and the term *mummy* itself are derived from *mumia*, the Latin word for

Introduction

asphalt. Use of the corpses themselves arose from confusion between the methods of preservation and the mummies themselves. Astonishingly, mummia was included in the 1924 price list of Merck & Co, the pharmaceutical company founded in the seventeenth century and now a multinational concern. Although the *wound man* (see frontispiece) is a common figure in mediaeval medical books, it remains true that for centuries little if anything could be done about the majority of such injuries. Many, if not most, of those injured would have succumbed to haemorrhage before complex operative surgery, or infection before antibiotics. Inevitably there is no evidence of soft tissue injury in the archaeological record but we know that for centuries those who were injured in conflict received scant if any care unless they were worthy of ransom, and upon their death were stripped, pillaged of any possessions worth taking and confined to mass unmarked graves.

The commonest cause of death following trauma is bleeding and although control of external bleeding by use of a tourniquet or pressure has been possible for centuries, it inevitably required the advent of effective surgery to treat bleeding from internal organs. As we shall see, the importance of a simple means of controlling bleeding in order to save lives is a lesson the medical profession has had to relearn repeatedly: a penny that did not finally drop until the end of the twentieth century, although tourniquets were used during Alexander the Great's Campaigns and by the Roman

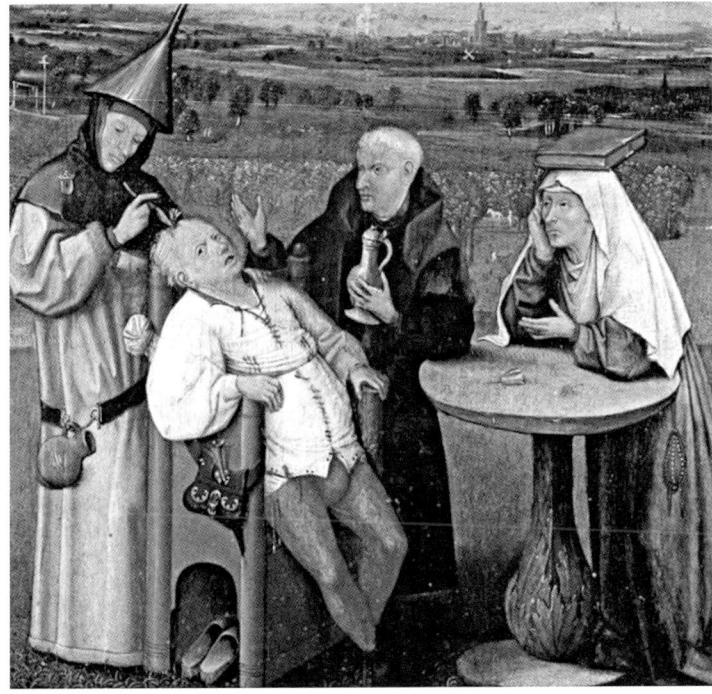

Trepanning;
*a painting by
Hieronymous Bosch.*

Army. Similarly, until the late nineteenth century limb trauma was commonly treated by amputation which was one of the few surgical procedures simple enough and quick enough to be carried out without anaesthetic. Prosthetics (artificial body parts) have been around since ancient times – the ancient Egyptians did a neat line in artificial toes – but in truth, little if any progress had been made into early modern times.

Upper limb replacements tended to be cosmetic rather than functional, although devices incorporating knives and hooks were common, and lower limbs at first did little more than stop the wearer falling over. When the Marquess of Anglesey lost his leg at Waterloo in 1815, the artificial limb with which he was fitted was one of the first with a reasonably effective knee joint and it was only during the nineteenth century that any attempt at realistic motion in a false leg was made.

Although the Syrian Arab physicians and Saints Cosmos and Damien are said to have carried out a leg transplant in the third century CE, reimplantation surgery did not become a practical reality until the second half of the twentieth century.

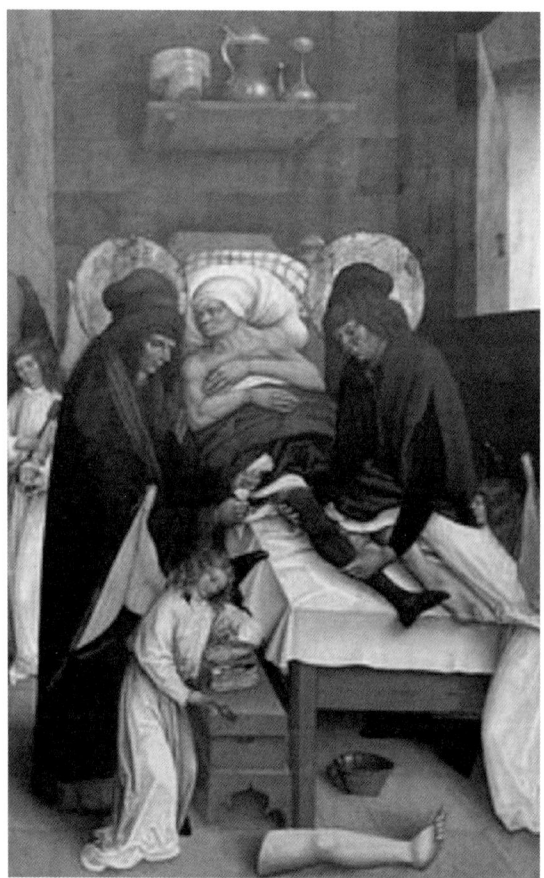

Saints Cosmos and Damien transplant a leg.

Introduction

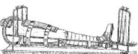

Thus, we reach the early 1800s with little sign of significant advance since ancient times. Surgery for internal trauma remains impossible and reconstructive surgery is only a dream. Amputation is the treatment for serious limb injury and is frequently fatal, carried out on a conscious patient with limited analgesia. Survival depends, as ever, on the skill of the surgeon and on serendipity. The distinguished surgeon Sir Robert Liston is said to have, on one occasion, amputated the patient's testicles as well as his leg and on another allegedly took off one of his assistant's fingers and slashed the coat of another. The second assistant died of shock and the first, together with the patient, of infection. Despite this tale of woe, stories of bones being broken over the operator's knee before amputation of a limb can be discarded. Infection post-surgery or post-trauma is widespread and the return to normal function uncommon. Antibiotics and antiseptics are unknown and infection with Dickens' *Ignorance* and *Want* stalks the wards as it stalks the slums of the burgeoning industrial cities. Medical care for the poor, always those most at risk of injury, where it is provided at all, relies on charity and the voluntary efforts of surgeons relying on the guineas of the wealthy for their livelihood.

The scene is now set and we can turn our attention to Birmingham on the eve of the industrial and manufacturing explosion of the first decades of the nineteenth century.

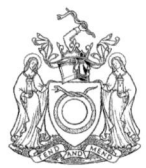

Prelude

Temple Row, Birmingham 1825

IMAGINE A SMALL but vibrant market town about the size that Stevenage, Hartlepool or Grimsby are today. A smart modern church by the go-to architect of the day stands at its heart and streets of modern classical houses are gradually spreading in rows of disciplined elegance outwards into its ancient quarters. Activity: trade, philosophy, science, social intercourse and industry are all enthusiastically engaged in by its citizens. The railway has yet to reach Birmingham and transform it, but within five years the politician William Huskisson will become known as the first person to die following a railway accident, his leg mangled by Stephenson's Rocket on its inaugural run on the Liverpool to Manchester railway. Amputation not being possible, he will die later the same day. (In fact, 13 year-old John Bruce had died under the wheels of a locomotive in Leeds in 1813, prompting the no-nonsense *Leeds Mercury* to comment that the incident would "operate as a warning to others." He was almost certainly the first railway fatality and one of the early casualties of the industrial revolution which was soon to engulf Birmingham.)

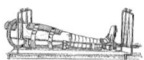

A tall gentleman, the term gentleman is important, walks along Temple Row, the town's fashionable medical quarter, near to St Phillip's Church. He is expensively, if plainly, dressed with a high forehead and hair which is a little long and fails to do as he wishes, especially when he is excited, as he is now. He carries a sheaf of papers, a

Prelude

vague air of moral superiority and a sense of purpose. He is William Sands Cox, aged 24 and a significant person in a small town which is awkwardly on the verge of its nineteenth century expansion.

Early nineteenth-century Birmingham is at a point of transformation; a vibrant community with a sense of its own potential, breaking free from its ancient status as the hub of a rural economy and prosperous market town and increasingly dominated by men of ideas. Matthew Boulton and James Watt the engineering pioneers, Erasmus Darwin physician and writer on evolution, Richard Lovell Edgeworth the novelist, Samuel Galton Jr., arms manufacturer, Joseph Priestley discoverer of oxygen and the potter and anti-slavery campaigner Josiah Wedgwood, have all made their impression on the town. Sands Cox, like his town, is conscious of a sense of possibility limited only by lack of ambition and is motivated by a commitment to hard graft.

Birmingham's first steam train will arrive in 1837. Reason and experiment, and a profound belief in progress have replaced superstition, acquiescence and unquestioning social deference. The town's luminaries who meet by the light of a full moon and call themselves *lunaticks*, members of the Lunar Society, have created the Birmingham enlightenment and the town is a vibrant and exciting place to be. There is inevitably tension between the old ideas and new ways of thinking: Priestley would end his life in America after his laboratory was burnt down by a mob outraged at his support for the revolutionary movements then sweeping Europe.

St Phillip's Church will not become a cathedral until 1905 and the town is still relatively small with a population of 90,000 people in 15,000 homes. Within 75 years Birmingham will have a population of half a million; a teaming industrial city, canal and railway hub, the place where plastic is first created and the home of the first postal service; but for now, as Sands Cox approaches the most important meeting of his life, it is a small but bustling market town with aspirations. *Drake's Picture of Birmingham: intended for the use of residents and visitors* published in 1830 describes a town still bounded by landed estates with fingers of agricultural land poking into its heart, but with evidence of burgeoning industrialisation.

Near the church stands the parsonage and Blue Coat School, and not far away a Quaker meeting house built in 1707. Early signs of developing industrial greatness can be discerned in the many small workshops making buttons, nails, buckles and jewellery and nearby stand the grand houses of the professional and entrepreneurial classes. Matthew Boulton's pioneering Soho "manufactory" stands separate from the town across open fields. The town also has an increasing sense of civic pride and a desire to improve the lives of its citizens. Neat Georgian houses in smart terraces four storeys high with bright classical doorcases approached by gleaming steps and windows in regimented rows enclose the land around the town's new church.

The "Acci"

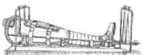

Surgeons are only of late gaining professional status compared to physicians, graduates of the ancient universities, holders of degrees. The old saw *"physicians at the front door, surgeons round the back"* is less heard than it used to be. Increasing professional recognition is gradually putting clear water between surgeons and tradesmen. Although a surgeon, William Sands Cox is definitely a gentleman. Born in Birmingham on 19th May 1801, the son of Edward Townsend Cox, surgeon to the town's Workhouse, Dispensary and Garrison Hospital and educated at the town's already famous King Edward's School, he now lives with his father in one of those fine houses overlooking the churchyard. Edward Townsend Cox, his *British Medical Journal* obituary of 1863 remarked, *"settled at Stratford on Avon; but, finding a country life more to his taste, he shortly removed to Birmingham."* William had been born at 38 Cannon Street of a family long established in the area of Stratford-upon-Avon, Warwickshire.

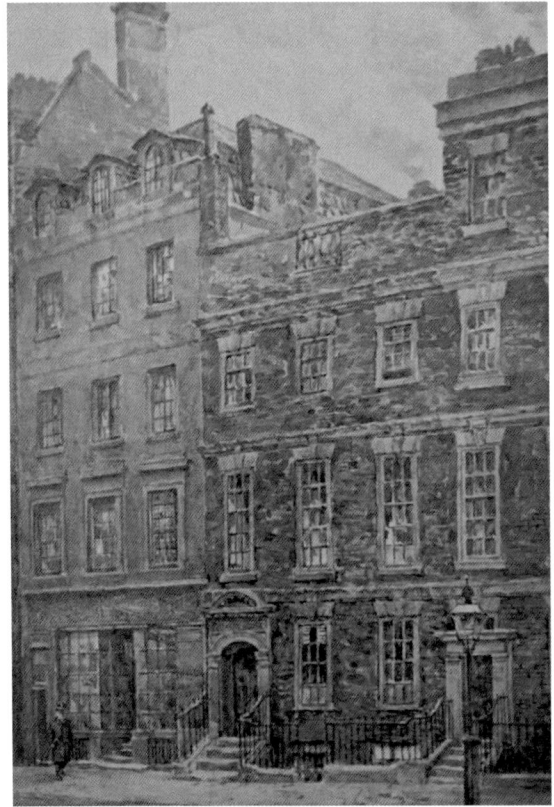

Mr Sands Cox's House, 24 Temple Row.

Prelude

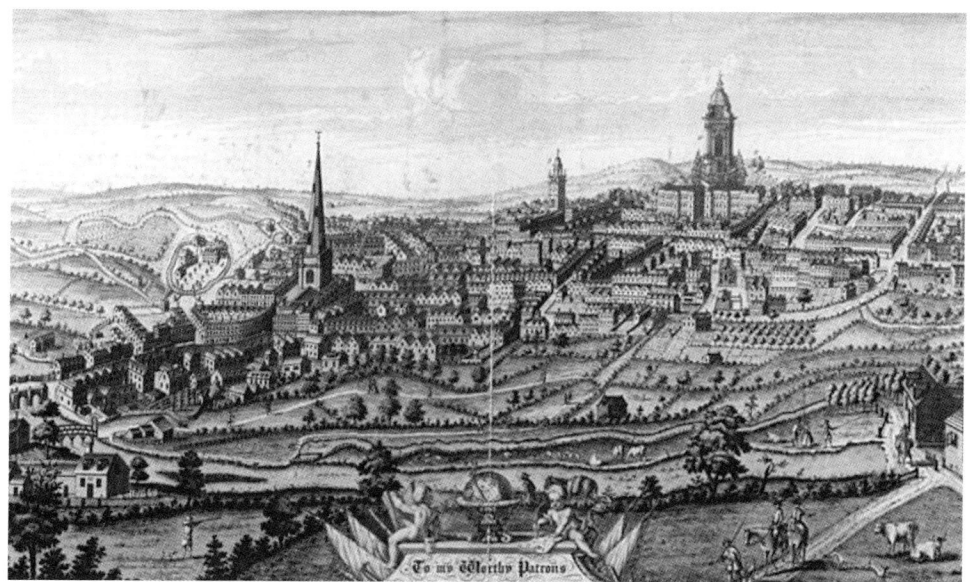

Birmingham, 1832, St Phillip's Church is on the skyline to the right.

Originally intended for the Church and then apprenticed to his father, (his indenture survives in Birmingham's striking new library) Sands Cox had moved to St Thomas' and Guy's Hospital in London where he was apprenticed to Sir Astley Cooper (the most eminent surgeon of the day, surgeon to the King and a friend of Sands Cox's father). He had been admitted to the Society of Apothecaries in 1823 and to the Royal College of Surgeons in 1824, before returning to his home city after gaining experience in Paris, doubtless making the most of his father's established practice and reputation.

A later visitor arriving uninvited at William Sands Cox's house would describe his *"miser-like face, tangled hair and scrubby beard"* and slovenly dress, noting that he had *"evidently hurried from his bedroom without the customary ablutions"*. Every square foot of surface of his study *"floor, chairs, tables, shelves and every other coign* [projecting corner or angle of a wall] *of vantage"* was *"piled up with books, reports, law papers, printers' proofs and other literary matter, begrimed with dust and apparently in the most hopeless condition of muddle."* Surprised by his unexpected visitor, Sands Cox asked for an hour to prepare himself to receive guests and on reacquaintance, his visitor found him *"in a soberly cut coat of black, a brilliant black satin waistcoat, and white necktie* [looking] *as he always did in this dress like a well to do English country clergyman."* At dinner parties where ladies were present he was described as very quiet, but with a *"merry twinkle in his eye"* when the conversation became animated.

Today, as he returns to his father's house after taking coffee, with a copy of the *Birmingham Gazette* under his arm and a bundle of manuscript notes in his hand, he has great things in mind: he is to found a medical school. Shocked by the drunken and licentious behaviour of the medical students in London, a theme to which we will return, he has been inspired to establish a medical school in Birmingham where students can be protected from the temptations of the metropolis and better encouraged in diligent study and Godly behaviour. Medical students have been informally taught in the town before, including by the first surgeon to the workhouse, John Tomlinson, but this is something different.

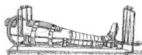

Sands Cox's grand scheme begins modestly with a series of lectures delivered by him in his father's house, but progress is rapid. Lecturers are appointed and the school is formally recognised in 1828, moving to a smart new building where Snow Hill Station now stands, in 1834. In 1836, a group of local worthies submit a memorandum to King William IV, and His Majesty is graciously pleased to become patron of the school which was to be styled the Royal School of Medicine and Surgery in Birmingham, an accolade enjoyed only by Birmingham and Manchester medical schools.

There is something of the puritan about Sands Cox and after his medical school becomes part of Queen's College in 1843, there is a split which leads to the theological faculty separating from all the other subjects and becoming Queen's Theological College. The other subjects form Mason Science College and in 1900 this becomes the University of Birmingham.

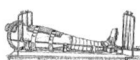

Medical students need patients to practise on, and although Sands Cox is a welcome sight on the wards of Birmingham's venerable General Hospital, spurred on by his earlier success, it is not long before he has embarked on his second great campaign.

Birmingham needs another hospital where medical students can be exposed to disease and injury and absorb the wisdom of their superiors. Founded in 1765 by local worthies, including Matthew Boulton, John Baskerville, the printing type designer and printer to Cambridge University and Sir Lister Holte of Aston Hall, the General Hospital looks more like a stately home than a place for treating the sick. It has three floors and nine windows on each floor on the main front, the middle three projecting forwards a little under a pediment. The central main entrance is classical and approached by balustraded steps. The sides are shorter, but plain and absolutely

Prelude

symmetrical. The basement is half hidden below ground and the top floor windows are shorter and square as they might be in any smart contemporary mansion. There is a lower wing on each side. Part of the wave of new hospitals that included Guy's in London in 1725, St George's, also in London, in 1733 and Edinburgh Royal Infirmary in 1736, the General Hospital is, like them, built on the twin foundations of scientific enquiry and commercial prosperity. However, after its promoters run out of money, at least in part due to transferring their funds to the construction of the new Birmingham Canal, it finds itself funded from the proceeds of a triennial music festival where performances of Handel's *Messiah* regularly raise large sums of money and which continue to fund the hospital until the twentieth century.

The General Hospital's most famous physician, well known to Sands Cox, is William Withering, physician, member of the Lunar Society and the first to describe the use of digitalis in heart failure. Its first treasurers are the button maker John Taylor and Quaker iron master Sampson Lloyd who have set up a banking business in Dale End, which will eventually become Lloyd's Bank. Unfortunately, the new hospital only has 40 beds, and refuses to allow access to Sands Cox's students as it has its own paying private students. The infirmary wing of the nearby municipal workhouse built a century before offers some opportunities for clinical observation, but not nearly enough to support the students of a flourishing and growing medical school.

With his reputation for probity, commitment and getting things done, Sands Cox launches his appeal for his new hospital in 1839 and such are his powers of persuasion,

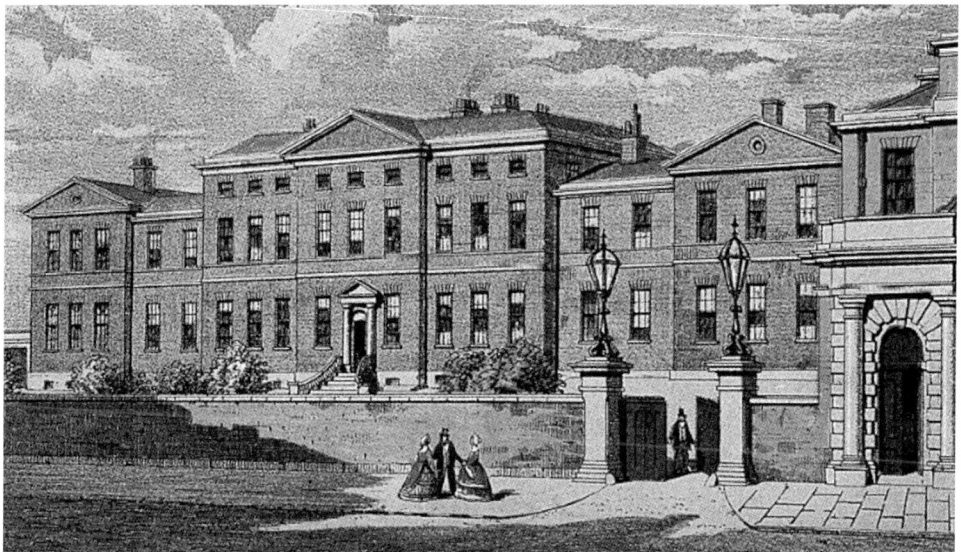

Birmingham General Hospital.

reaches his target the following year. A donation of £200 is received from the Rev Samuel Warneford who later becomes a regular and generous benefactor to the school and hospital, but is in part responsible for the later split of Queen's College, of which he is also a benefactor, due to his uncompromising Anglicanism. A shy, weak vicar's son who grew up to marry into wealth, the adult Warneford, also in holy orders, was reclusive. His wife died insane three years after their marriage leaving him extremely wealthy. Unusually for the time he refused to commit her to an asylum and nursed her at home until her death; he never remarried. His clothes were old-fashioned, his house dirty and shambolic, his meals frugal and although he travelled long distances to keep a watchful eye on his benefactions, the horses which pulled his carriage were bought for a song at the end of their working lives. Warneford's generosity to numerous causes, including Birmingham's Hospital was matched by a religious intolerance amounting to bigotry. His final words as he lay dying would be, "*I should have been kinder, I should have been more considerate and understanding.*" He was particularly concerned about the morals of medical students, commenting, "*What is said about the absorbing nature of a medical student's pursuits is but too true, and it is one of the evils which most requires remedy, it is this which narrows their minds and makes them bigots to low infidel views*". He certainly knew a thing or two about narrow minds, but despite his reservations, or perhaps because of them, he funded churches, missionary societies, education for the orphans of clergy, and hospitals and medical schools including the Radcliffe Infirmary in Oxford, Kings College in London and, most importantly for our story, Birmingham's new medical school. However generous his largess was elsewhere, charity definitely did not begin at home, his importuning family saw none of it and were described as hoping for "*detested Samuel's demise*".

As might be expected, Warneford insists that the new medical school is exclusively Anglican. His donation stipulates the appointment of a Church of England chaplain who is to be paid £40 per annum. As a consequence, perhaps, the hospital has two chaplains from when it opens its doors until the day it closes. Proving that not much changes in the world of building, Sands Cox's builders go bust, but unsurprisingly its determined originator purchases the necessary materials himself and for six months pays the workmen's wages out of his own pocket, a measure both of his commitment and his professional success. The building is completed free from debt on 18th June 1841.

The new hospital costs £935 15s. At the time, a farm labourer earned £30 a year, one of Birmingham's skilled artisans perhaps £75 and a doctor, though not our own Sands Cox, around £200. The social standing of physicians was much higher than today, at least in part due to their status as gentlemen, and as late as 1925 the Centenary History of the Birmingham Medical School included adverts for Buicks, Chevrolets, Daimlers and Rolls Royces, doubtless suitable for visiting one's paying patients.

Prelude

(Telephone: Midland 3040 *"We wish to assure intending purchasers that their enquiries by letter or by a visit to our Show Rooms will not result in constant calls from Salesmen, which we know cause considerable annoyance."*) In the heat of the country's industrial expansion an engineer or surveyor might on average earn two and a half times as much as a surgeon. The foundation stone of the new building is laid by Earl Howe on 18th June 1840 and a glass vase containing coins and medals is embedded under the stone. The ceremony is preceded by a public breakfast in the town hall attended by 450 people. A Masonic procession led by the mayor, with music provided by the band of the Royal Scots Greys, proceeds from the Town Hall to Bath Row, where the hospital stands. More than 10,000 people watch the stone being laid. The site chosen for the new hospital is described as the most elevated, open and salubrious westward of the town. It has fields in front of it and looks across the *"field path to Edgbaston"* to open countryside beyond; a salubrious place for the ill and injured. Nearby stands the Worcester Canal Office and St Thomas' Church. In a moment of justifiable pride, Sands Cox opens the hospital himself in 1841. Like her predecessor, Queen Victoria grants her patronage to the new teaching hospital and allows it to be styled "The Queen's Hospital", a privilege unique to Birmingham's new building. The hospital's first president is Prince Albert the Prince Consort, symbol of the triumph of science over superstition and founder of the Great Exhibition. It is possible that her association with the new hospital is prompted by her horror at the working lives of the Midland's industrial poor. Queen Victoria may even be the first person to have coined the term "Black Country", she certainly wrote in her diary in 1832, *"the country is very desolate everywhere; there are coals about, and the grass is quite blasted and black. I just now see an extraordinary building flaming with fire. The country continues black, engines flaming, coals, in abundance, everywhere, smoking and burning coal heaps, intermingled with wretched huts and carts and little ragged children."*

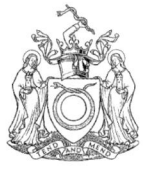

Chapter 1

Foundations

SANDS COX'S NEW hospital was the first hospital outside London to be built specifically for the teaching of medical students. Nurses at the time were not formally trained and were generally considered to be of the status of domestic servants of the lowest sort. In *Martin Chuzzlewit* (1843) Dickens would caricature contemporary nurses in the drunken, incompetent and umbrella-wielding Mrs Gamp, based on a real-life example described to him by the Victorian philanthropist Angela Burdett-Coutts. Until the University of Birmingham was founded in 1900 by amalgamating Queen's College and Mason Science College as the first English "red brick" university to receive its own Royal Charter, students had to do part of their training in London in order to have their qualification recognised by the Royal College of Surgeons and Society of Apothecaries and thus be awarded their degrees.

It is difficult after the passage of almost two centuries to imagine the life of a nineteenth-century medical student. There is no doubt that in pre-anaesthetic, pre-antibiotic days, before treatments began to be subjected to rigorous scientific assessment, many therapies were equally brutal and ineffective. The presence of pus in a wound was considered a healthy sign of healing and referred to as *laudible pus* and there was no real understanding of the causes of infection. Students were as susceptible as patients to these diseases and learning medicine carried a significant mortality. Many diseases were considered to be caused by contaminated air, the *miasma* theory of disease, until, in 1854, John Snow, a London general practitioner and pioneer anaesthetist proved beyond reasonable doubt that cholera was spread by contaminated water. Noticing that cholera cases were much more common amongst those who gained their drinking water from a specific street pump, Snow simply removed the pump's handle and observed the consequent reduction in cases and deaths as people used alternative sources for their drinking water. This simple, but provocative action not only saved many lives directly and indirectly, but also established the science of epidemiology and the speciality of public health. Snow and others like him, including Birmingham's William Withering with his careful investigations into the use of digitalis from foxgloves for heart disease, were early pioneers of a new medicine built on scientific foundations, in the establishment of which the Birmingham Hospital would play a major part. If the new medical students at the Queen's Hospital would be amongst the first to benefit from the belated emergence of physical medicine from its long hibernation, they would continue to learn little about the care of those with psychiatric conditions. Although there had been significant improvements since the second half of the eighteenth century, largely as a result of the pioneering work of Quaker reformers, there was still a long way to go and mental ill-health bore a stigma which to some extent it still retains. When the great poet of the English countryside John Clare died in 1863, his cause of death was given as *"years of poetical prosing"*. There was, however, some recognition that the mentally ill should be treated with kindness, even if no specific therapies were available. At least the more histrionic were no longer a source of Sunday afternoon entertainment for polite society. However, as Sands Cox's hospital establishes itself, the medical student still faces a life of crushingly hard work, long hours, heavy alcohol consumption and indoctrination with methods which were often crude, regularly dangerous and not infrequently fatal. Medical students 100 years later were told *"half of what we teach you is wrong, the problem is, we don't know which half,"* this was spectacularly the case in the mid-nineteenth century. It is perhaps unsurprising that nineteenth-century medical students acquired an unsavoury reputation.

The development of the new hospital was rapid; the dispensary and home visiting department began work almost immediately and the first patients were admitted on 24th October 1841. Within only a few years of the hospital's opening, a new detached block containing 28 beds for patients with infectious disease was built, bringing the total number of beds to 98. The foundation stone of the new extension was laid on 16th July 1845 by William Sands Cox's proud father, Edward Townsend Cox.

From the start, the town (and later the city) and its people took the hospital to their heart. Benefactors, of which there were many, were recorded on marble tablets in the new hospital. Sadly, these plaques were removed when the hospital closed and have since been lost. The artisans of Birmingham gave £905 5s 6d derived from penny subscriptions in 1847 and £1,070 13s 3d was raised from a concert given by Jenny Lind, the *"Swedish*

1. Foundations

Nightingale" and the most famous soprano of her day, in the Town Hall on 28th December 1848; (*"The Committee of Council* [of the Queen's Hospital] *have the pleasure to announce that Mademoiselle Jenny Lind having generously offered her gratuitous services in aid of the above charity, A GRAND CONCERT WILL TAKE PLACE IN THE TOWN HALL"*). The advert, unsurprisingly, was signed by William Sands Cox and tickets cost from one pound one shilling (reserved) to five shillings standing. In 1856 a half share of £5,054 12s 4d was raised from two fêtes held at Aston Hall and organised by manufacturers and tradesmen. An annual ball was established *"under the patronage of the nobility and gentry of the town and midland district"*, although one suspects that Sands Cox himself was not a natural party-goer. All these figures can be multiplied by around 70 to give their true purchasing power today. In 1859 Sands Cox launched an appeal to collect one million penny postage stamps, the following year he was able to report in the press that enough stamps had been received to *"erect two additional wings, comprising wards for diseases of women and children, for burns and accidents of a similar character, for diseases of the eye, and a chapel and to extend the outpatient department"*.

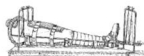

As we have already seen, the middle and late nineteenth centuries were a time of transformation in medicine. Eighteenth-century medical men were almost as likely to put you out of your misery, as cure you, and in the case of surgery the cure, such as it was, as well as the complications were frequently worse than the disease. Before the first use of surgical anaesthesia in Britain in 1846, the patient's only hopes were manual dexterity and speed. Robert Liston, who we have already met in charge of the only operation in medical history with a 300% mortality, was incidentally also the first surgeon to carry out an operation under anaesthesia when he amputated Frederick Churchill's leg through the thigh. Pre-anaesthetic surgery was crude and rapid, not because surgeons wanted it to be, but because there was no alternative if the patient was to stand a chance of survival. The widespread acceptance of anaesthesia was remarkably rapid, probably aided by Queen Victoria's use of chloroform during the birth of her eighth child Prince Leopold in 1853. She described it as *"blessed chloroform, soothing, quieting and delightful beyond measure"*. In fact, there was considerable resistance to the use of chloroform in childbirth as it was believed that the pain of delivery was, as one (inevitably male) obstetrician put it, part of the *"natural and physiological forces that the Divinity has ordained us to enjoy or suffer."* Anaesthesia entered military use within a short time of its discovery, Russian surgeon Nikolay Ivanovich Pirogov using ether as an anaesthetic in 1847. He was also the first surgeon to use anaesthesia in a field operation during the Crimean War.

Anaesthesia brought about a solution to one of surgery's most important problems, but it was not until 1865 when Joseph Lister introduced antisepsis that the curse of post-surgical infection, septicaemia and death was finally challenged. Thereafter longer and more complex procedures became possible and practical modern surgery was born. At the same time, physicians such as Sands Cox's friend William Withering were developing the practice of medicine based on careful observation of natural phenomena and the detailed analysis of the results of their actions, underpinned by scientific advances uncoupled from religion or established dogma. Withering's achievement was not that he recognised that foxglove extract was an effective treatment for dropsy, oedema caused by retention of water in the tissues, as it had been used as a folk remedy for generations, but rather that he established what the key ingredient was and demonstrated its effectiveness by a series of controlled clinical trials which he published in *An Account of the Foxglove and some of its Medical Uses* in 1785. Equally importantly, with his fellow members of the Lunar Society and William Sands Cox and others, he was a driving force in Birmingham's enlightenment.

Queen's Hospital produced its own pioneers as part of the nineteenth-century leap forward in medicine and surgery. Augustus Volnay Waller (1816-1870), and his son Augustus Désiré Waller (1856-1922) were distinguished physiologists and were part of the first generation to attempt to understand how the human body works at a cellular level. Augustus père was a physician and professor of physiology who described the degeneration of divided nerves which now bears his name and is known as Wallerian degeneration. A fellow of the Royal Society at 35, he also made important discoveries concerning the function of blood cells. His stay in Birmingham was brief and he retired to St Leonards-on-Sea to study sea urchins before carrying out medical practice and research in Paris, Bruges, and Geneva. Ever the practical man, and a martyr to seasickness, he wrote that on a journey to London on the Ostend ferry he *"found nausea already commencing. Pressure on the vagus* [nerve] *produced sleep on two occasions, and I was able to escape the enemy"*. Definitely not something to be tried at home.

The nineteenth century was also the period during which the medical profession became organised, regulated and professionalised. Balthazar Walter Foster (1840-1913) studied medicine at Trinity College, Dublin. After graduation, he taught anatomy at the Royal College of Surgeons in Ireland, but decided not to pursue a medical career, applying instead for a commission in the Royal Navy. Despite this he was appointed demonstrator in practical anatomy at Queen's College Birmingham in 1860 and professor of medicine in 1868. He described the medical community in Birmingham as having a *"new atmosphere of modern thought and scientific enterprise"* compared to the traditionalism of medicine in his home city of Dublin. By this time a well-established researcher, he was the first clinician in England to publish a paper on premature death from ketoacidosis among diabetics. A pioneer in the treatment of tuberculosis, in 1870 he published *Method and Medicine*, a defence of scientific research as the foundation of clinical medicine. In 1885 he was elected member of Parliament for Chester as a Liberal candidate on a ticket advocating free education and improved housing for the poor. He was a strong supporter of Joseph Chamberlain's campaign to improve Birmingham's sanitation and a typical representative of Birmingham's liberal and intellectual elite. The first doctor to hold a ministerial post in Britain, Foster organised the national sanitation campaign between 1892 and 1895, which successfully prevented the 1893 cholera epidemic reaching Britain. He was responsible for the direct representation of the medical profession by election to the GMC and in 1910 was elevated to the peerage, as *Baron Ilkeston* of Ilkeston in the County of Derby.

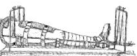

It is all too easy to assume that the relatively simple procedures which are important elements of modern medicine have been hallowed by centuries of use. In truth, very few treatments which are still in use predate the nineteenth century and many that we take for granted were introduced only recently. Sampson Gamgee (1828-1886), a giant (no pun intended) amongst Victorian surgeons, although now largely forgotten, was surgeon at the Queen's Hospital from 1857. As a young man he had shared lodgings with Joseph Lister and like Lister he was a pioneer of antiseptic surgery. Having served as a surgeon in the Crimean War, on his return he introduced cotton wool as a surgical dressing; combined with surgical gauze it was known as the Gamgee bandage and if applied by an expert took on the nature of a splint. Gamgee also invented the disposable sanitary towel and introduced plaster of Paris splinting of fractures to Great Britain. In 1873 Gamgee founded what is now the Birmingham Hospital Saturday Fund (commonly known as the BHSF) but was originally known as the "Working Men's Fund for the Extension of the Queen's Hospital".

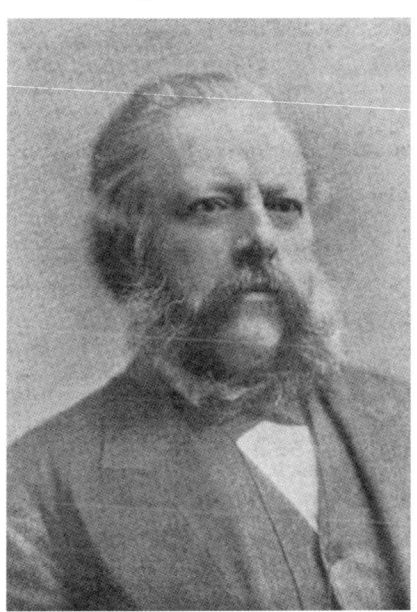

Sam Gamgee: surgical pioneer and proto-hobbit.

Gamgee's oddest claim to fame has nothing to do with his medical practice: he gave his name to the hobbit Sam Gamgee in J.R.R. Tolkien's *The Lord of the Rings*. Tolkien grew up in Birmingham after his father's death and like Sands Cox before him attended King Edward's School.

There is no doubt that the Queen's Hospital was a powerhouse in the scientific transformation of medicine. Its other early clinicians who were pioneering in their own fields included Furneaux Jordan (1830-1911), a surgeon who devised an operation for amputation of the leg at the hip and Jordan Lloyd (1854-1913), professor of surgery, who wrote about the surgical treatment of gunshot wounds to the abdomen and neck, various fractures and the management of wounds to the major blood vessels.

Perhaps the greatest and most important (especially in view of the subsequent establishment of the Accident Hospital) of these Victorian clinicians was Dr John Hall Edwards (1858-1926) who, inspired by the work of Roentgen and also a life-long passion for photography, built an X-ray machine at the Queen's Hospital. Edwards was a Birmingham boy through and through, having been educated at King Edward's School and qualified in medicine at Queen's College.

On 11th January 1896, Hall took an X-ray of a colleague's hand in order to locate a needle. This is believed to be the first recorded medical use of X-rays. A month later, on 14th February he took the first radiograph used to plan a surgical operation. In 1899 Edwards was appointed surgeon radiographer, the first such post in the World and effectively the forerunner of every one of today's radiologists. During the Boer War he established the first ever field radiology service, writing a series of letters for the *Birmingham Daily Post* describing his experiences. By 1904, X-ray induced malignancy in his left arm caused Edwards to be the first person to describe X-ray burns in humans with the result that safety measures began to be put in place to render medical use of X-rays safe. His left arm was amputated in 1908 and he later lost some of the fingers of his right hand. His left hand is preserved in the Birmingham University Anatomical Museum as a specimen illustrating malignant change due to radiation (specimen 01.1135.1!). As a result of his occupational damage Edwards was granted a pension of £120 a year by King Edward VII. His interest in photography led to work debunking the so-called spirit photographs which were popular after the First World War; he was particularly critical of Sir Arthur Conan Doyle's gullibility in accepting the so-called Cottingley Fairies as genuine. Like several of his colleagues, a pioneer in public health, and having done much to promote knowledge of cancer in the medical field, Edwards died of cancer induced by radiation in 1926.

As the nineteenth century progressed, the Queen's Hospital continued to grow. In 1862, the outpatient room was enlarged and two new wards and a chapel were built.

1. Foundations

The cost of £1,600 was raised from Sands Cox's penny postage stamps. In 1867 the house and grounds of St Martin's Rectory next door were purchased in order to build a new outpatient department and nurses' home. Gamgee's Working Men's Fund for the Extension of the Queen's Hospital with additional contributions, raised enough for the building work and the foundation stone for the outpatient department was laid on 4th December 1871 by Lord Leigh. The enthusiasm and generosity of the people was astonishing, especially given the low wages of nineteenth-century industrial workers, and it in turn inspired Queen Victoria to contribute £100 to the institution named after her. Some years earlier she had donated to the hospital a copy of Winterhalter's portrait of herself.

Originally designed simply to fund the hospital extension, Gamgee's fund perhaps inevitably became a permanent way for Birmingham's hospitals to raise money. Its main source of income would come from overtime earnings given by workers on nominated *Hospital Saturdays* when they worked an extra shift. The first such fund to raise money in this way for multiple hospitals, it was another manifestation of the close relationship between the burgeoning working classes of industrialising Birmingham and their hospitals. On the chosen Saturday, street collections continued to be made to support the hospital's work. It has been argued that Gamgee's fund was the germ from which health insurance developed and it has even been suggested, a little hyperbolically, that it was a step on the way to the idea of a National Health Service. When Gamgee established his fund, it joined the already existing annual *Hospital Sunday*, itself the brainchild of the Vicar of St Martin in the Bullring when all the money collected at church services was earmarked for the town's hospitals. His idea of involving the working classes of Birmingham directly in the funding of their hospital was one of genius. By 1938 many of the working people of Birmingham were making small regular contributions and £275,000 was raised which was the main financial support of all Birmingham voluntary hospitals.

On the first official *Hospital Saturday*, 15th March 1873, more than £4,000 was raised through street collections and from workers who donated earnings from working overtime on that day. From 1878, instead of a single day of collection, workers were invited to contribute a penny a week from their wages, leading to annual donations of £10,000 or more. Few British hospitals were as embedded in and well supported by the communities they served: a link that would survive until closure. In 1891 the Hospital Saturday Fund became a "not-for-profit" company able to buy land and property for use as convalescent homes. The first home opened at Tyn-Y-Coed near Llandudno in 1892, and its facilities were available to all men living within five miles of Birmingham Town Hall. Here the men could spend a couple of weeks in gentle exercise and relaxation before the return trip to the city. Two years later a similar home, also in Llandudno, was opened for women, followed by a third for children. During the Second World War the construction workers of the floating Mulberry Harbours used in the Allied invasion of Normandy in June 1944 would be housed at Tyn-Y-Coed. Other homes followed in Great Barr and the Lickey Hills, Malvern and Weston-super-Mare, though only the one in Weston-super-Mare survives today. The fund also provided home nursing, surgical appliances and artificial limbs. In 1895 the city's horse-drawn ambulance service was supplemented by four special ambulances designed to deliver an injured person more swiftly and comfortably from the scene of an accident to hospital; the first of many initiatives that would follow in improving the care of the injured before they reached hospital. The Birmingham Hospital Saturday Fund still survives as a not-for profit health insurance provider more commonly known as BHSF.

When the hospital extension was opened by the Mayor of Birmingham, Ambrose Biggs on 7th November 1873, a thousand children from the Birmingham Schools' Choral Union sang a hymn written for the occasion by the Revd Charles Kingsley, author of *The Water babies* and the historical novel *Westward Ho!* called *From Thee All Skill and Science Flow*. Kingsley is now most famous, if famous at all, for his novels but he was equally known during his lifetime as a social reformer, especially concerned about child welfare. He was also a friend and correspondent of Charles Darwin whose shocking theory of Evolution he supported. The resort in Devon, Westward Ho! is named after Kingsley's novel and is simultaneously the only place in England to be named after a novel and to have an exclamation mark in its name.

This new extension was known locally as "The Workman's Extension" and was designed by the local architects Martin & Chamberlain, architects of more than 40 of Birmingham's board schools, which were part of the town's growing social conscience, civic pride and collective confidence.

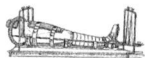

William Sands Cox, founder of Birmingham's medical school and the Queen's Hospital died in December 1875 at the age of 73. In 1831 he had published his great work *Synopsis of the Bones, Ligaments and Muscles, Blood-vessels, and Nerves of the Human Body* and in 1836 he had been elected a Fellow of the Royal Society; an unusual honour for a surgeon. In 1857 £1,050 was raised by public subscription as a testimonial to Sands Cox, which he devoted to founding scholarships and to completing the museums of Queen's College.

In 1860 the Charity Commission carried out an investigation into the management of the hospital and medical school with the result that the two

1. Foundations

> TESTIMONIAL TO WILLIAM SANDS COX, Esq., F.R.S.—At a MEETING of the Friends of WILLIAM SANDS COX, Esq., F.R.S, held at QUEEN'S COLLEGE, BIRMINGHAM, December 15, 1856,
>
> JOHN RATCLIFF, Esq., the Mayor, in the Chair,
>
> It was resolved,
>
> That Mr. Sands Cox having devoted his life to the establishment of the Queen's College and the Queen's Hospital, at Birmingham, both of which Institutions have now, by the blessing of God, proved their stability and their great value to the town and district, that means be taken for evincing the appreciation in which such disinterested devotion of time and talent is held by the public, and that in furtherance of that object contributions be solicited from the Nobility and Gentry, the Commercial and Manufacturing Interests, and Artisans of the town and Midland district.
>
> It was further resolved,
>
> That the following Gentlemen do form a Committee for effecting the above object, with power to add to their number:—John Ratcliff, Mayor of Birmingham, Chairman; James Thomas Law, Chancellor of the Diocese of Lichfield, Vice-chairman; Mr. Edward Armfield, Thomas Bagnall, Esq., Mr. James Busby, Mr. John Boucher, Mr. Morris Banks, John Birt Davies, Esq., M.D., Mr. Samuel Haines, Mr. Phillip Harris, Mr. Samuel Hemming, Mr. William H. Osborn, Mr. Jacob Phillips, Mr. John B. Payn, Mr. John Suckling, Hon. Sec.; Mr. James Shaw, Mr. G. Taylor, Treasurer; Frederick I. Welch, Esq, Mr. Thomas Upfill.
>
> JOHN RATCLIFF, Mayor, Chairman.
>
> Contributions will be received by every member of the Committee, and by all the Birmingham Banks.
>
> JOHN SUCKLING, Hon. Sec.
>
> 35, Cherry-street.

Testimonial to William Sands Cox, Staffordshire Advertiser, *27th December 1857.*

institutions were separated. The Royal College of Surgeons biography of Sands Cox comments in a rather disappointed tone, *"it appears his administrative ability was not equal to his creative power and he became embroiled in serious quarrels with his associates"*. The tribulations of Sands Cox's foundations were aired in great detail in the local papers with complaints of significant debts, failed endowments, declining use by the public and teaching salaries unpaid. The *Birmingham Daily Post* published a letter from the Dean of the Faculty of Queen's College to the College's visitor, the Bishop of Worcester, stating, *"I complain of the arbitrary, tyrannical and overbearing conduct of Professor W Sands Cox, towards all who presume to differ from him in opinion, as well as of his complete inefficiency in every office which he now holds in the College and Hospital, and I pray your Lordship to avert the impending destruction of these institutions by at once removing him therefrom"*.

It would appear that Sands Cox, as the Founder of his two institutions developed a near obsession with their daily management and like many creative people was unable to recognise the need to hand over to a younger generation. An assessment written after his death commented that *"his mind was creative only…and had always been wanting in the sustaining power which successfully carries on great work, he insisted* upon regulating every matter of detail and discipline connected with the two institutions". A sad end to a distinguished career.

Perhaps unsurprisingly, the Dean's letter and the publication of the Charity Commissioners' report verbatim in the paper resulted in legal action for libel by Sands Cox. Once the legal matters were finally dealt with, and the investigation was behind him, Sands Cox took no further part in the running of either institution. Feeling *"disappointed, dispirited and dejected"*, he left Birmingham after his father died in 1863 and lived first near Tamworth, at Leamington, and finally at Glass House, Kenilworth, where he died. He was buried at Aston Parish Church, Birmingham. The published report of his funeral noted that *"during his lifetime Mr Cox [sic] held strong views on the absurdity of many prevailing funeral customs, and his interment on Friday week was carried out in strict conformity with the instructions left by the deceased...He expressed a wish that if he should die in England he might be buried in the family vault within the Aston churchyard; that his body might be conveyed there in a plain hearse, without plumes or any decorations whatever, and carried from the gates to the vault by six old medical students of Queen's College, Birmingham."* A puritan to the last.

It is difficult after the passage of time to gain a true feel for Sands Cox's obviously complex personality. He is described as having *"few amusements. He was fond of a quiet rubber [of bridge]; he kept a tame monkey whose grotesque antics were to him a constant source of amusement. With fly rod he was very skilful"*. On one occasion, having forgotten his own box of bait, he simply stuffed a handful of worms in the pocket of his waistcoat. A posthumous tribute comments that his apparent miserliness concealed an essential generosity and kindness of heart. He clearly also had a certain charisma, *"there was something marvellous in the power he possessed of influencing others."* His genius was for turning ideas into reality and for encouraging those around him to support them; usually by putting their hand in their pocket. There is no doubt that he was a challenging colleague and a poor manager, but there can equally be no doubt that through his devotion to the citizens of Birmingham and the Midlands, Sands Cox had earned a place in the hearts of the people and an enviable reputation as a surgeon across the nation; his testimonial was reported in the London papers and a notice of his death was printed in papers as far away from Birmingham as Dundee. Sands Cox left little in his will to the two institutions he founded, perhaps due to the Commissioners' report and a lingering sense of bitterness at the way he felt he had been treated, but one suspects a wry smile as he left sufficient money for *"defraying the expense of continuing the publication of accounts of the Queen's College and Queen's Hospital"*. He left his books, instruments, microscope, £3,000 and *"the chair in which King Charles I sat during his trial in Westminster Hall"* to Moreton-in-Marsh Cottage hospital, £3,000 for the building and endowment of a church in Balsall Heath and

£12,000 for the building of three dispensaries. He also bequeathed money for the establishment of medical scholarships at King Edward's School and Guy's Hospital. He left a wife, Isabella, but there is no evidence of any children.

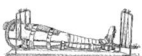

A medical facility that Birmingham could be proud of was embedded in the generosity of its citizens, many of them poor, supported by the aristocracy and the town's intellectual and industrial elites and staffed by clinicians of national reputation. In 1875, Queen's Hospital became a free hospital, abandoning the previous system whereby the hospital's financial supporters issued "subscriber's tickets" to authorise treatment. An admission fee of one shilling was charged but could be waived if the patient was unable to afford to pay it. In 1877, 16,117 patients were treated at the Queen's, but by 1908, the annual number of patients had more than doubled to 39,483, including 2,685 inpatients and 36,708 outpatients. Treating this number of patients was expensive and the hospital's average annual expenditure from 1909 to 1911 was £14,729, against average receipts of £10,778, leaving an annual deficit of £3,951 which was covered by endowments and donations. The nurses' home was built in 1887 to accommodate 38 nurses and the two original wings were extended at the same time.

Electric lighting was installed in 1889 at a time when domestic electricity was the preserve of the wealthy. In 1900, William Humble Ward, 2nd Earl of Dudley, friend of Edward VII, owner of more than 200 coal mines, numerous steel works and more than 30,000 acres of Shropshire and Worcestershire, took over the presidency of the hospital. A new block opened in 1908 with three storeys of wards. The nursing home's capacity increased to 74 beds, and the hospital itself now had 60 medical and 118 surgical beds. The hospital's number of beds continued to increase until it finally closed.

More ground to the west of the hospital was purchased in 1904 and a large medical block was opened. On 23rd October 1908, a new chapel was built. The last major development consisting of six surgical wards and three operating theatres was built between 1925 and 1927.

During the First World War the Queen's Hospital treated British and Belgian soldiers. William Billington, appointed consultant surgeon at the Queen's Hospital in 1913, was posted to the military 1st Southern General Hospital, established within Birmingham University at the outbreak of war where he was put in charge of treating jaw and facial injuries. By 1918 the 1st Southern had more than 6,000 beds. Few people can have imagined that in only 20 years staff from the Queen's Hospital would again be treating the wounded from another world conflict. After the Great War, many voluntary hospitals struggled financially. Support came in the form of a government grant which was administered by the Voluntary Hospitals Committee which later became part of the Birmingham Hospitals Council. The Council was responsible for the co-ordination of appeals for money, the development of local hospitals in relation to one another, the collection of information about the needs of hospitals and their patients and facilitating co-operation between hospitals. In many ways it was the forerunner of local and regional health authorities that were established as part of the National Health Service after 1948.

In the 1920s Dr Stanley Barnes, a neurologist at the General, and later Dean of the Faculty of Medicine, suggested the possibility of building a new medical school adjacent to the University in Edgbaston with a new hospital adjacent to it, replacing the Queen's and General hospitals in the city centre. The medical school and new hospital, named the Queen Elizabeth Hospital after Queen Elizabeth, later Queen Elizabeth the Queen Mother, were built on land donated by the Cadbury family, wealthy from the public's passion for confectionary, builders of Bournville model village and benefactors of the city. This new development was the last great achievement in the city of the voluntary hospital system before it was replaced by the development of the National Health Service. The first beds opened in 1938, but as a result of the outbreak of World War II the plan to close the Queen's Hospital failed to materialise and it remained open, albeit with fewer beds.

When the Queen's Hospital's future looked most bleak with the opening of the new Queen Elizabeth Hospital nearby, a group of Birmingham businessmen decided that the old hospital still had much to offer. The close relationship between the old hospital, the population of Birmingham and the city's industrial elite came to its rescue. Fortuitously for the hospital, and with war looking more probable, a number of prominent people in and around Birmingham, particularly those involved in industry, became very interested in setting up a better method of treating the injured, particularly those involved in industrial accidents. The driving intellect behind this initiative was Dr Donald Stewart, a local industrial medical officer, who, together with the Association of Industrial Medical Officers and the University of Birmingham were actively interested in improving the facilities for the treatment of the injured. A committee was formed, which brought together representatives from the Queen Elizabeth, Queen's and General hospitals, the great and good of Birmingham and the medical school and met to look to the future management of casualties as the international situation continued to deteriorate and a second World War, only 20 years after the close of the first, appeared increasingly likely.

Mr Keats of Pressed Steel (later British Leyland) represented Birmingham's manufacturing industry. Other important figures were Dr Matthew Burn and Sydney

1. Foundations

Vernon, a Birmingham solicitor and later Pro-Chancellor of the University of Birmingham. At the same time, it had become clear at a national level that the treatment of the injured by Britain's hospitals was so poor that in 1939 the government appointed a committee of enquiry to visit all the hospitals in England and report on the standards of trauma treatment and recommend changes necessary to improve those standards. The committee published their report in 1939 as *The Rehabilitation of Persons Injured by Accident*. In response to this report and to local pressure the University agreed to lease the Queen's Hospital at a peppercorn rent. With all the stars aligned, in 1941 the Queen's Hospital would become the Birmingham Accident Hospital, known across the city as *The Acci* and it was the World's first trauma centre.

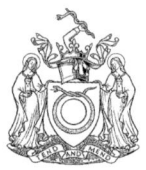

Chapter 2

A Hospital at War

THE TRAUMA SYSTEMS and centres that have transformed trauma care across the UK in the last decade, largely came into existence as a result of a series of highly critical reviews of trauma care across decades when there was little if any improvement in treatment of the injured and the engagement and interest of consultants and hospital managers was limited. Such reports, as we have seen, are nothing new. It was the earliest of these *The Rehabilitation of Person's Injured by Accident* report of 1939 which led to the creation of the Accident Hospital, combined as it was with high levels of trauma in a major industrial city and the potential for devastating effects of future German bombing. It was ultimately the War which led to the establishment of Birmingham's own centre of excellence for the treatment of victims of trauma and its international reputation. Half a century later it would be later wars, in Iraq and Afghanistan, that would thrust Birmingham again to the forefront of trauma medicine.

One of the most important findings of the 1939 report, and a situation that persisted into the 1980s, was that most patients with injuries were treated by junior and inexperienced doctors, or if they were really unlucky, medical students. The more established consultants were occasionally heard to remark in a rather superior manner that the victims of trauma were poor, smelled bad, were often drunk and obnoxious and prone to arriving at hospital at socially inconvenient times, 24 hour care was a rarity and treatment often unacceptably delayed as a consequence. In addition, before the onset of more generous social provision, patient follow-up required time off work and consequently loss of pay, with the result that those who needed it most were often

2. A Hospital at War

least able to obtain it. Occupational health services were still poorly developed and treatment, when it was available, was not informed by expert knowledge of industrial conditions.

As a result of the establishment of a committee to look into trauma care in Birmingham, Dr Matthew Burn, Deputy Medical Officer of Health for the city, agreed to visit the distinguished Bohler Clinic in Vienna and information was sought regarding the number of casualties arising each year from the industrial plants of the Midland counties. The Austrian orthopaedic surgeon Lorenz Bohler is widely considered to be the father of European trauma surgery. He had learned advanced surgical skills in the United States and honed them during his service in the First World War. On his return to Europe he had approached the AUVU – the labourers' accident insurance organisation (snappily known as the *Arbeiterunfallversicherungsanstalt*) and with its support opened his country's first accident clinic in 1925. His clinic was an obvious destination for anyone wishing to improve the care of the injured.

Thus everything was in place for the "Queen's" to become a trauma hospital. The outbreak of war inevitably caused a delay, but in February 1940 when it was becoming clear that the casualties of war were likely to be added to those of industry, Professor Parsons, on behalf of the United Hospitals, organised a conference on casualty services and Sydney Vernon explained how the Hospitals Council wanted to retain the Queen's Hospital for the treatment of the injured. It was remarked that the hospital was in a pleasant area on the edge of the city centre which was (wrongly, as we shall see) thought to be safer in time of war. A committee was set up to establish the provisional Board of Management for what was initially called the *Fracture Hospital* and remarkably, it was agreed that if the successful candidate for clinical director was serving in the Armed Forces, they would be released. A request was also made for a grant from the Ministry of Health to help with the setting up of the new hospital. The first meeting of the Provisional Board of Management of the new hospital took place in December 1940. It was agreed that the name would be the Birmingham Accident Hospital and Rehabilitation Centre. The emphasis on rehabilitation was both pioneering and important, even to this day trauma services in the NHS provide a level of rehabilitation services which most experts consider inadequate. Given its subsequent workload, the medical staff of the hospital was remarkably small consisting only of the clinical director and senior surgeon and his deputy, an assistant surgeon, two anaesthetists, a surgeon in training and four surgical house officers. During its first nine months in operation the bill for medical staff salaries was £950 2s 0d (for nursing staff £2,091 6s 0d, the whole hospital budget was only £33,279 18s 0d).

The "Acci"

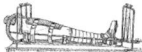

The Birmingham Accident Hospital (BAH) opened on 1st April 1941. By this time, every priority of Birmingham's industry and every aspect of the lives of its population were devoted to the prosecution of the War against Nazi Germany. Now a major industrial centre, and a city since 1889, Birmingham's factories produced Spitfires and Lancaster bombers, military vehicles, aircraft components, engines and small arms. Like many manufacturing centres, Birmingham was heavily bombed: the Birmingham Blitz began on 9th August 1940 and ended almost three years later on 23rd April 1943. Hospitals were, of course not immune. City hospitals were particularly vulnerable to air raids. On 23rd November 1940, Sister Galloway and Sister Daniels who had just finished their shift at the Royal Orthopaedic Hospital were killed instantly when bombs fell on the building. A further incendiary bomb was extinguished by Sister Hyden. On 18th November 1940, what was still at that time the Queen's Hospital would itself be hit by incendiary bombs. Leslie Phillips, a 26-year-old assistant in the hospital's laboratory, was dealing with an incendiary bomb in the hospital grounds when he saw another land on the roof of the medical block. Climbing to the roof accompanied by two firemen and then sliding down a sloping roof alone, Phillips extinguished the fire using buckets of sand passed to him by the firemen before using a stirrup pump to dampen down roof timbers to stop the fire from spreading. Phillips would receive a civilian gallantry award on the recommendation of the hospital's House Governor who commented that his action had "*saved the hospital from very severe damage*".

During the course of the Birmingham Blitz 2,241 people were killed and 3,010 more seriously injured; 3,682 people sustained minor injuries. Almost 2,000 tons of bombs were dropped in 77 raids, making Birmingham the third most heavily bombed city in the United Kingdom after London and Liverpool. Although targets such as the Spitfire factory in Castle Bromwich were destroyed, most of the destruction rained down on residential and commercial areas. As well as 300 factories and almost 250 other buildings, more than 12,000 houses would be destroyed and many more damaged. The first raid on the city centre was on the night of 25th August 1940 when the Market Hall in the Bull Ring was destroyed and the Birmingham Small Arms (BSA) factory, which produced barrels and machine guns, was first damaged.

Damage to water mains meant that the city's fire services had to obtain water from the canals to extinguish fires started by incendiary bombs. Public transport was interrupted by damage to the city's tram network. Gas supplies and sewers were also damaged. Determined to carry on, the city arranged a meals service for workers at bomb-damaged factories.

Similar raids took place across the industrial Black Country, fortunately with relatively limited loss of life, but extensive damage to industrial areas in Dudley, Wolverhampton, West Bromwich, Smethwick and elsewhere.

During the course of the Birmingham Blitz, German bombing destroyed 12,391 houses, 302 factories and 239 other buildings in the city; hundreds of others were damaged, thousands of citizens were made homeless. Birmingham University, City Art Gallery, Town Hall and the Council House were severely damaged as was St Philip's Cathedral (St Phillip's Church had become a cathedral in 1905) which suffered serious fire damage after being hit by an incendiary bomb. Fortunately, its glorious stained glass by Edward Burne-Jones had been removed for safety. St Thomas' Church, on Bath Row, a stone's throw from the Queen's Hospital was largely destroyed on the 11th December 1940, leaving only its portico and tower. The gardens surrounding it were later dedicated as a peace garden.

The raids were particularly heavy in November 1940 when 800 people were killed and 2,345 injured; 20,000 civilians lost their homes. Many factories were badly damaged including Lucas Industries, GEC and the Birmingham Small Arms Company for a second time. On this occasion 53 employees were killed and 89 were

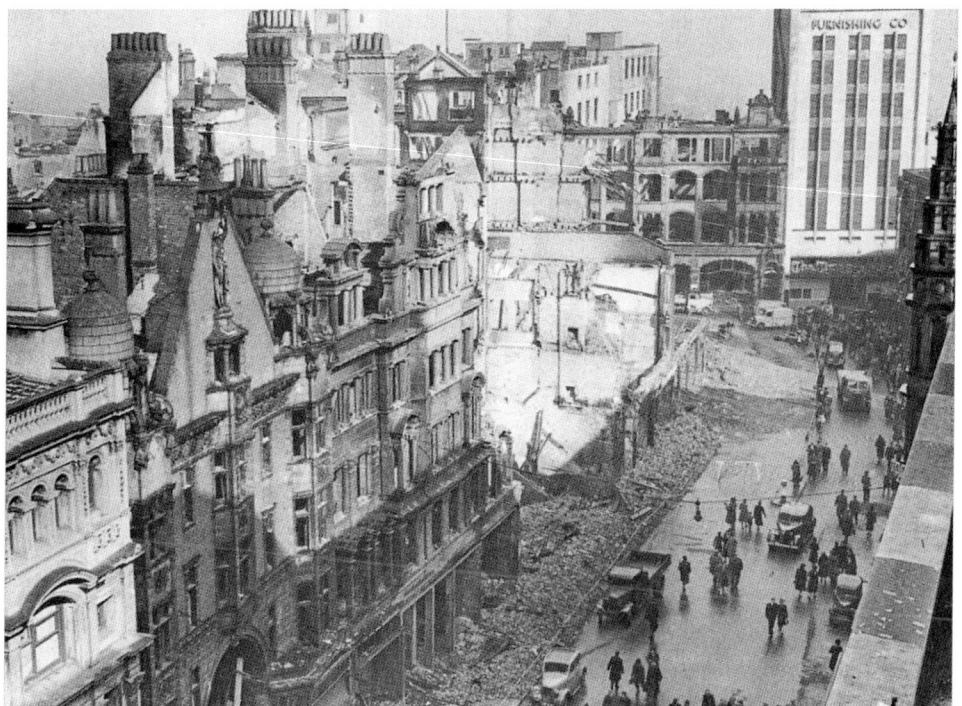

New Street after a German raid.

injured. From early 1941 major raids targeted the city centre rather than industrial sites and considerable damage was caused, not only to iconic buildings such as St Martin's Church in the Bull Ring, but also to the poorer inner city residential areas that surrounded the commercial and civic centre. This then was the situation in which the Queen's Hospital and subsequently the Accident Hospital, found itself in the early years of the War. Fortunately, as so often happens in such times, a man of vision and capability was on hand to turn a desperate situation into an advantageous one and to cement even further the relationship between his hospital and the people of the city. His name was William Gissane and he was appointed by the governing body to be director of the new hospital and its senior surgeon.

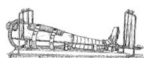

William Gissane, who is in many ways the hero of this story, was a sports-mad Australian, passionate about golf, cricket and rugby. An appreciation late in his life commented that he *"lived his early life in an athletic atmosphere"*. Born in Sydney in 1898 he had been captain of his school cricket and boxing teams and played rugby for the public schools of New South Wales before service in the Royal Australian Artillery during World War I. He studied medicine at the University of Sydney where he won blues for both cricket and boxing and became light heavyweight inter-university champion.

Gissane graduated in 1925 and that same year left for England, working his passage as the ship's surgeon on SS *Ataka Maru*; his interest in trauma surgery began during a period of work in London and was reinforced by time spent in Vienna working under Bohler's supervision. The lessons he learnt in Vienna were not lost on the enthusiastic Gissane who would dedicate his working life to the service of the injured.

Aside from the immediate problems presented by the Blitz, which threatened to overwhelm the city's hospitals, there were the ever-present and all too frequent injuries in heavy industry and manufacturing where maintaining output was essential and health and safety legislation limited. Many experienced male staff had been

> **VESSELS IN PORT.**
> **AT PORT ADELAIDE..**
> Alpena, 4-m. sch., 833, Johnson, from Raymond. Walter & Morris, agents. Corporation Wharf. (Discharging timber.)
> Ataka Maru, 2,481, Watanape, from Port Pirie. George Wills & Co., agents. Big Crane Wharf. (Loading.)

From the Adelaide Register, December 1915.

called up for military service and were replaced by less experienced female employees. Bombed-out buildings, the blackout (and driving in the dark) and high levels of poverty only added to the potential workload. Despite all these risks, the Birmingham Accident Hospital was the only specialist trauma hospital to open in Great Britain during the War and the only specialist trauma centre to open until a second centre opened in Stoke-on-Trent more than 40 years later. It was also the last voluntary hospital to open before the advent of the National Health Service and at first had no endowments, investments, or a public subscription list. It relied entirely on the promises made by industry and individual donors for financial support. Curiously, wartime regulations made it illegal to publish the names of the hospital's donors.

A man from the same mould as Sands Cox, but with an undoubtedly greater ability to manage as well as innovate, Gissane's drive and organisational ability as director and surgeon in chief soon transformed the old Queen's Hospital into the new Accident Hospital. Throughout his professional life he would practice in accordance with three fundamental principles: separate the sick from the injured, ensure that appropriate personnel and facilities for treatment and investigation are immediately available for the injured – senior surgeons should be on the spot or a short distance away on call; there should be no waiting for X-ray or theatres and finally, care of the patient should be in the hands of the same clinical team from arrival through to rehabilitation and discharge. Within a very short period of his arrival, Gissane would be able to attract the country's best burns specialists to realise his desire to establish the area's first specialist Burns Unit.

In the years that followed he would be a pioneer, not only in the treatment of the victims of trauma, but also in establishing the world-leading Burns Unit at the BAH of which he was appointed surgeon-in-chief. Until the day of its closure, the BAH remained an international centre of excellence in burns management. As part of a team, including Leonard Colebrook as director of the MRC Burns Research Unit and others such as Ashley Miles, Robert Williams, John Bull, Edward Lowbury and later Ruscoe Clarke, Douglas Jackson and Simon Sevitt, he led what was referred to as the "Birmingham experiment" in patient care. His work on the reduction of road and industrial accidents brought him international recognition. He was made CBE in 1964 and was awarded an honorary doctorate of science from the University of Wales and a life membership of the British Association of Plastic Surgeons. His interest in accidents and their consequences brought him into contact with industrial processes and machinery and especially the motor industry, where the work of clinicians at the Accident Hospital had considerable influence on efforts to address car safety issues. In 1961 Birmingham University made him an honorary professor of accident surgery, the World's first such appointment. Fittingly, Gissane died in his sleep on 1st April 1981 – the 40th anniversary of the establishment of the Birmingham Accident Hospital.

Gissane brought with him to Birmingham Dr Joe Wolfson who had been a colleague at St James's Hospital in London and was chosen by him to be the BAH's first senior anaesthetist after military service during the War. In his book, *Anaesthesia for the Injured* Wolfson commented *"It is the author's opinion that concentrated experience of anaesthesia for trauma (including burns) in accident centres, which are likely to become established throughout the country in the future should become part of the training of all anaesthetists"* and *"... the anaesthetist can usefully become a fully integrated member of the team treating injured patients, not only in the operating theatres, but in the management of respiratory and circulatory problems, in resuscitation, in the relief of pain, and in a number of diagnostic and therapeutic procedures in which the techniques can be helpful."*

Wolfson was an early advocate of massive blood transfusion for the critically injured and of avoiding the use of anaesthetic agents which caused loss of blood pressure and exacerbated shock in the injured. His vision of trauma centres across the United Kingdom would not be achieved in his lifetime.

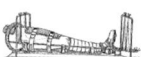

As the conflict intensified, the unique response of the Accident Hospital developed. Unsurprisingly, the number of people injured also increased dramatically. As well as the casualties of the bombing, with increased levels of war-related activity, during 1940 and 1941 the number of industrial injuries in the Birmingham area requiring treatment at one of the city's hospitals increased by at least 40%, the annual total now being well over 100,000.

In response to the challenges of the War, the hospital provided a 24 hour a day service with continuous cover, including a consultant surgeon available at any time of need, 24 hour X-ray capability, blood transfusion and most unusually a mobile operating theatre based at the hospital but capable of travelling to where it was most needed. Of these innovations, in retrospect the most important would be the 24 hour availability of a consultant, something recommended in reports on trauma management as late as the early twenty-first century and certainly unique in 1941 and for decades afterwards.

When the Accident Hospital opened, the Queen Elizabeth and General Hospitals (the United Birmingham Hospitals) provided the buildings and made no charge for the contents and medical equipment which were left for the Accident

2. A Hospital at War

Hospital's use. It was agreed that any donations, grants and endowments received by the original Queen's Hospital be transferred to the new United Hospital and that if or when the Accident Hospital closed, the buildings and land would revert to the United Hospitals. It was a condition of the hospital's establishment and consistent with the founding function of the "Queen's" that its staffing was to be sufficient for the teaching of medical students. As a result, generations of Birmingham medical students would gain clinical experience much sooner in their careers than would even be thought possible by their modern successors. When the handover occurred, a small midwifery department remained and use of outpatients was retained by the United Hospitals until alternative arrangements could be made.

In 1941, the new hospital had 322 fully equipped beds, of which 83 on the top floors could not be used during the War by direction of the Ministry of Health, presumably due to the risk air raids. Of the available beds, 50 were reserved for the injured victims of air raids, leaving 189 for the use of other injured patients. Beds were available for injured men, women and children, all strictly segregated according to the custom of the time and generally preferred by patients today, whatever social engineers might say to the contrary. The number of beds reserved for air raid victims would fall after the Battle of Britain and the lessening of the threat from the air, but in 1942 it was noted that 22 of the women's beds were occupied by male battle casualties, the women having been moved elsewhere.

On 22nd June, 16 days after D-Day, the first of 11 convoys brought injured soldiers to the by then well-established Birmingham Accident Hospital, and in total the hospital treated 183 battle casualties some of whom remained as inpatients for more than six months. At the end of the War, 194 beds were in use.

As the War progressed and the Hospital's war work increased, its outpatient department, built and opened in the 1870s, became increasingly unsuitable and plans were made to rebuild it. Wartime constraints meant that this would require a building licence from the government, which inevitably had other things on its collective mind, and work was delayed. The new department would not, in the end, open until 1944 but when it did, its provisions were in advance of anything then available.

The new department consisted of a reception department with a resuscitation room, reception cubicles, three operating theatres and X-ray suites as well as an outpatient treatment department with consulting rooms, a plaster room and further X-ray facilities in addition to a soft tissue dressing area. Each area was designed for efficiency and to allow the maximum number of patients to be treated by the minimum numbers of staff. At the dedication service, Charles Kingsley's hymn, composed for and sung at the opening of the Queen's Hospital outpatient department in 1873, was sung again.

The hospital's patients were divided into three groups: fractures and serious injuries, injuries not involving bone but including infections and finally, rehabilitation patients. This emphasis on the rehabilitation of the injured was, as we have seen, in itself pioneering. Previously, victims of trauma were discharged as soon as they were fit to leave hospital and largely left to fend for themselves. Those injured during their work were generally unable to take time off and either returned before their recovery was complete, or fell into the limited provision then available for the unemployed.

A brief look at the finances of the new hospital will give an indication of the small scale of the hospital in the early 1940s. In 1941 the hospital's total income was £26,791 10s 5d, just over a million pounds in today's values. Industry contributed £10,009, the city of Birmingham £5,000 and the Ministry of Health £7,249. The Birmingham Hospitals Contributory Association contributed £3,320. The Contributory Association had been launched in 1928 and in conjunction with St John Ambulance also began operating ambulances to improve the carriage of patients to the city's hospitals. The ambulance fleet initially had a paid staff consisting of a driver-mechanic, two drivers, one driver-orderly and two night and one day ambulance sisters. By 1938, in time for the outbreak of war, the service had 15 vehicles. Contributors to the Association were charged 2s 6d per journey, the normal fee being 9d per mile (return), with a minimum fee of 10s.

Returning to the hospital; coal, gas, and electricity cost a total of £1,566, nursing staff £2,091 and medical staff £950 10s 4d (only £34,000 in today's terms). Mr Hugh Carson was acting clinical director and was supported by temporary assistant surgeons F.G. Allan, H. Donovan, and T.S. Donovan. Miss M.J. Rowley was on the staff as an anaesthetist and William Gissane started on 1st September as surgeon in chief and clinical director. L.J. Wolfson started as senior anaesthetist on 17th November. Despite the available expertise, when necessary the treatment of brain and abdominal injuries would be supported by surgeons from the United Birmingham Hospitals. The junior medical staff consisted of one resident surgical officer, one resident surgical registrar and house surgeons.

In the first year of its existence the hospital treated an average of 110 inpatients and 350 outpatients each week, including significant numbers of air raid victims. Their average length of stay was 13 days. Miscellaneous expenses included a pharmacy cost of £11 for wines and spirits, probably largely bed time "tots" and stout, which was believed to have health promoting effects due to its high iron content and was available in Birmingham's hospitals until the 1990s. Another notable entry in the extraordinary expenditure account was for £294 for the hospital's photographic room. There was still a need to raise capital for building projects and funds were raised by a capital appeal and a broadcast appeal by the Mayor of Birmingham. The relationship

2. A Hospital at War

with Birmingham's industry remained close as one industrialist remarked, *"you tell us what you need and leave us to find the money"*.

Donors were able to endow a bed for £1,500, a not-insubstantial sum equivalent to £60,000 in 2020 terms. There were no takers for this generous offer and in 1943 the fee was reduced to £1,250 leading to the Birmingham Small Arms Company providing an endowment; in 1945 the General Electricity Company Bed was dedicated. In 1944 as a result of funds received from the Ministry of Health for the treatment of battle casualties, the hospital astonishingly had an excess of £653 income over expenditure. As casualty numbers increased, the clinical challenges became greater because the government placed a limit on the number of staff allowed to work on the "home front". With troops fighting to contain enemy advances across three continents, the Central Medical War Committee unsurprisingly maintained that their priority was to appoint medial staff to look after the fighting services.

By 1943 the Accident Hospital was seeing more than 20,000 patients a year with limited staff, under the most difficult of circumstances. As the tide of the War turned, around 10% of patients were serving members of the Armed Forces.

The special challenges of the War led to two pioneering appointments. In 1942 Dr J. Rhaiadr Jones became the hospital's first rehabilitation consultant; one of the earliest such appointments in Britain, and in 1945, in response to the prevailing patterns of wartime injuries, Colonel Leonard Colebrook was appointed to head the Medical Research Council (MRC) Burns Unit with a team of junior staff. In time this unit would be recognised as a world leader in the management of burn injury. The unit was established in two converted Nightingale wards and by the following year had four wards, each of eight beds together with a shock room, investigation room and treatment room with specially designed ventilation to reduce infection. There was also a saline bath annex. In their annual report, the hospital board wrote at length about the difficulties caused by junior staff being called up at short notice; inevitably it became difficult or impossible to maintain the team ethos established by Gissane.

Even after the Allied victory in 1945, there was no let up for the overworked clinicians of the BAH, indeed their particular expertise was recognised with an increasing number of roles; in almost every case working on areas of medical and nursing practice which had been neglected or ignored when the demands of war had focussed minds and the particular skills and experience of Accident Hospital staff had been elsewhere.

These developments resulted in the establishment of three "trauma teams", each led by a consultant with his own dedicated junior staff, an arrangement which survived, remarkably, until the hospital closed and was recreated in its new home. In 1946 J.R. Squire was appointed the director of the new MRC Industrial Injuries Unit supported by Betty Topley as research assistant. Amongst the important work this unit would perform would be pioneering studies of skin cancers caused by industrial exposure and research into the structure and function of the skin and the ways it responds to injury. Squire was also an early pioneer of computers in medicine and research.

As doctors returned from the fighting, the staffing of the BAH gradually reached more stable levels. New appointments included the remarkably named surgeon Peter Essex-Lopresti who had served with Airborne Forces during the War and whose paper *The Hazards of Parachuting* reported the injuries sustained by British Airborne Forces in 20,000 parachute jumps. In true BAH spirit, Essex-Lopresti recommended a number of actions to avoid injury, such as extending the neck to avoid hitting the forehead on exiting the plane and keeping the legs together when landing to prevent ankle injuries. He later received a Hunterian professorship from the Royal College of Surgeons, named for the most distinguished surgeon and anatomist of the eighteenth century, and is remembered to this day for the arm injury that bears his name. Essex-Lopresti died tragically young at the age of 35 in 1951.

Despite the large and growing workload, the staff of the now famous Accident Hospital remained small. There were four surgeons, four assistant surgeons, three surgical registrars and six house surgeons. Four anaesthetists and a rehabilitation specialist completed the front of house team. Behand the scenes, there was a team consisting of a pathologist, bacteriologist, radiologist, statistician (one of the first such appointments in a British hospital) and a team of researchers from the Medical Research Council (MRC) Industrial Medicine Research Unit. The MRC Burns Unit had a clinical director and three junior surgeons.

Dr John R. Rook joined the BAH as a consultant anaesthetist in 1947 or 1948. He published widely on trauma anaesthesia, was an advocate of careful pre-anaesthetic assessments and premedication, and drew attention to the risk of aspiration of stomach contents into the lungs during anaesthesia. Rook was also concerned about the risks of anaesthesia in the frail elderly and referred to the hazardous practice, then common, of dental anaesthesia with nitrous oxide ("laughing gas") as "dental asphyxia" or "surgical suffocation". He wrote *"In the Birmingham Accident Hospital, we believe that the drainage of a septic finger or the reduction of a Colles's fracture should be carried out carefully under the best possible operating conditions thus reducing the necessity for further operative procedures to a minimum"*.

When the hospital was first established, Miss E. Bullivant, the matron of the Queen's Hospital, agreed to stay on with a small nucleus of sisters. All the other nurses moved to the new Queen Elizabeth Hospital (QEH). As a result the new establishment's nursing staff were either trained nurses interested in specialist nursing of trauma victims or auxiliary members of the Civil Nursing Reserve. Newly qualified nurses could not be

2. A Hospital at War

recruited to the hospital. Throughout the War and after, nurses were trained at the Accident Hospital, working on the wards and in theatre after only two months of basic training. Members of the Friends (Quakers') Ambulance Unit acted as auxiliaries and helped with civil defence duties during air raids. As the War progressed, a number of local buildings were acquired or leased to provide accommodation for nursing staff; one such was still in use in the 1980s. Throughout the War years, around a dozen nurses passed their initial state examinations after training at the BAH. Only at the end of 1945 was the hospital allowed to recruit newly qualified State Registered Nurses (SRNs) but by this time two wards had closed due to lack of nursing staff.

As well as ministering to the needs of civilians and serving personnel injured as a result of war, the staff of the BAH continued its pioneering work in industrial health and safety, aided and encouraged by the hospital's strong links to local factories and manufacturers. In 1941 the hospital board in collaboration with the Royal College of Nursing, prepared a pioneering training course in industrial nursing with a certificate awarded by Birmingham University. Apart from the humanitarian need to avoid injury and death in the workplace, there was, of course, a need to maximise industrial output in aid of the War effort. In addition, there was a considerable overlap between industrial and war injuries. As we will see later, many of the widely accepted practices in civilian trauma care today continue to arise from the need to provide the best care for the victims of war.

Almost inevitably, with the vast and ongoing increases in industrial output, long hours, pressure to produce and massive influxes of new workers into manufacturing plants, arms factories, foundries and transport systems, accidents were frequent and of considerable concern to politicians focussed on prosecuting the war-effort. As late as 1945, comprehensive health and safety laws applied only to those working in mines and quarries and to a limited extent in factories, docks and shipyards, where they concentrated on the fencing, or guarding, of machines. In 1940, Rhys Davies MP questioned the Home Secretary Sir John Anderson about rising levels of industrial injury. The Birmingham course, the first of its kind, was therefore an important innovation. At the same time, training was offered to ambulance service personnel.

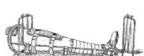

Just as the new courses in industrial nursing reflected Gissane's view of the importance of injuries in the workplace, so too did his drive to appoint medical officers to the Midland's large factories. The BAH would in due course appoint an industrial liaison officer, a mark of the remarkably close links between industry and the hospital. As a matter of routine, the new hospital would collect important data regarding treatment, rehabilitation and accident prevention which were shared with industrial medical officers. From the beginning, the Accident Hospital recognised the importance of effective treatment and rehabilitation for the victims of industrial and non-industrial accidents in returning them to their former status as wage earners and tax payers. This was, of course, especially important during wartime when there was an inevitable shortage of skilled workers due to the loss of those called up into the Armed Forces.

Thus from the hospital's inception, Gissane was committed to the importance of rehabilitation, a commitment reflected, as we have seen in the hospital's full title, the Birmingham Accident Hospital and Rehabilitation Centre. He is on record as saying, *"rehabilitation is an integral part of treatment and the title Birmingham Accident Hospital and Rehabilitation Centre signifies our intention to carry on the treatment of our patients until such time as they are fit to return to work."*

Recognising that a diet consisting solely of repeated physical exercise might be rather dull, and as a passionate advocate of effective rehabilitation, Gissane developed occupational therapy services to provide mental stimulus and enjoyable recreational therapy to increase engagement and commitment. These approaches were to be combined with traditional physio- and electrotherapy.

The novelty of this approach cannot be overemphasised and it is impossible to believe that Gissane and his colleagues were unaware of the pioneering work of Ludwig Guttmann at Stoke Mandeville. A brief digression about Guttmann is essential to any story of trauma care in the UK.

Born in 1899, Ludwig Guttmann (later Sir Ludwig Guttmann CBE FRS) was a neurologist and neurosurgeon who established the Stoke Mandeville Games, which evolved into the Paralympic Games. Banned as a Jew from practising neurosurgery in his university hospital, Guttmann became director of the Breslau Jewish Hospital where, following Kristallnacht in 1938, he defied the Gestapo by admitting injured jews and preventing their deportation. Before his own escape, he had developed an interest in spinal injuries after treating a coalminer with a broken back. In 1939, Guttmann was ordered by the Nazis to visit Portugal in order to treat the dictator Antonio Salazar. His return to Germany via London was interrupted by an offer to allow

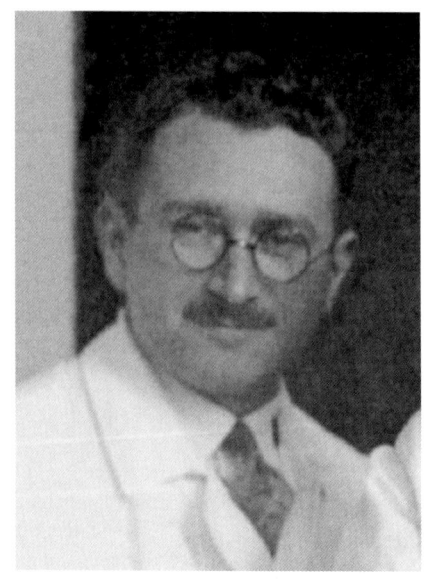

Sir Ludwig Guttmann.

him and his family to stay in Britain. He would become the founding father of organised multidisciplinary rehabilitation for the injured.

After his arrival in England, Guttmann continued his research in neurosurgery and became part of the vibrant community of refugee academic Jews in Oxford aided by a grant from the Council for Assisting Refugee Academics. It seems richly ironic that the Nazi's desire to rid mainland Europe of its Jews would so enrich the cultural and scientific lives of the countries in which those who were lucky enough to escape eventually settled. Guttmann's daughter would later become a friend of the actress Miriam Margolyes. In 1943, following an initiative from the RAF, keen to ensure the best treatment for their injured pilots, Guttmann established the National Spinal Injuries Centre at Stoke Mandeville Hospital in Buckinghamshire. He believed passionately that sport was an important method of therapy for the rehabilitation of injured military personnel. The first Stoke Mandeville Games would take place in 1948. Within a few years, the games established for injured veterans had become international and the first games alongside the Olympic Games were held in 1960. Guttmann became a British subject in 1945 and aside from his formal recognition, Guttmann, who died in 1980, received the unusual honour of appearing on a Russian stamp!

As we can see, Gissane based his approach to the injured on three fundamental principles: accident prevention, working with Birmingham's manufacturing industry and its medical staff, world-class treatment and multidisciplinary rehabilitation designed to return trauma victims to as near their former capacity as possible. These principles remain at the heart of effective trauma care.

Gissane predicted and passionately believed that the Accident Hospital model of integrated treatment and rehabilitation would be adopted by other hospitals throughout the UK. He would be astonished and disappointed to know that it took until the twenty-first century for a coherent network of specialist trauma hospitals to be established in the UK, and whilst pleased that advances in accident prevention have been dramatic and effective, would doubtless be astonished that there is still no effective consistent availability of rehabilitation services for the majority of trauma victims. It would be the surgeons in the USA who first established a network of trauma centres, although again, in the US and elsewhere, none of their trauma centres seem to have considered rehabilitation as an integral part of their role.

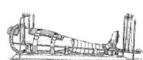

Despite the demands placed on a relatively small staff by the War and an ever-increasing workload, the need to raise funds remained a perennial problem and an additional burden for the staff and governors. In practice the hospital's status as Birmingham's own

"Acci" and the generosity of the city's citizens kept the hospital afloat. In 1941 a public fundraising campaign was considered but rejected because the medical staff were concerned it would attract more patients than they could possibly manage. In 1942 the Lord Mayor of Birmingham broadcast an appeal for funds and in 1943 a donation of two shillings from each factory worker was suggested. By 1944 the Lord Mayor's Appeal had reached its target of £20,000 and a second target to raise another £30,000 was launched.

In 1942, the Medical Research Council Wound Infection Unit was established at the BAH, led by two distinguished bacteriologists Professor (later Sir) Ashley Miles and Dr (later Sir) R.E. Williams. Bacteriologists study the causes and treatment of infections, then especially important, as the use of antibiotics was still in its infancy. Ashley Miles would become one of the most eminent bacteriologists of his generation. Amongst his achievements were pioneering work on wound infection and new techniques in counting bacteria, an apparently mundane technique which nonetheless allowed the seriousness of infections to be measured. Having served as sector pathologist for London he was appointed director of the MRC Infection Unit at the BAH in 1942 and served until 1946. Miles was also a member of the Medical Research Council, of the Public Health Laboratory Service Board and Committees of the World Health Organisation and was thus at the absolute heart of the early effective management of infection in the United Kingdom. He was elected a fellow of the Royal Society in 1961 and knighted in 1966. His wife, Lady Ashley, was the half-sister of the author Roald Dahl. At the BAH, Williams and Miles analysed the layout of dressing stations and developed a new system which was adopted by the hospital. They investigated the carriage of bacteria in noses and on skin and found that up to 50% of normal adults attending hospital carried the bacteria staphylococcus aureus in large numbers in their noses. Staphylococcus aureus was and remains a major cause of skin, and hence wound and bone, infections following trauma. One of the key members of Miles' and Williams' small staff was Dr Ethel Florey.

The discovery of penicillin is ascribed to Sir Alexander Fleming who noticed that fungal spores which had blown thorough his laboratory window at St Mary's Hospital in London had prevented the development of bacteria on a petri dish. Although Fleming later received the Nobel Prize for his discovery, difficulties associated with manufacturing penicillin in significant quantities meant that his eureka moment received little attention in the medical world until two Oxford scientists, Ernst Chain and Edward Abraham, began studying the molecular structure of the antibiotic, publishing their findings in 1940. Indeed, when Fleming telephoned Howard Florey, Chain's head of department, to say that he would like to visit the laboratory, Chain remarked, "*Good God! I thought he was dead.*" Within a relatively short time, Florey and Chain would transform penicillin from a laboratory curiosity into a useable drug which would save countless lives as the War progressed.

2. A Hospital at War

An Australian like Gissane, Howard Florey came to Britain on a Rhodes Scholarship. He worked first in London where he met and married Ethel Reed who would later bring some of the earliest trials of penicillin to the Birmingham Accident Hospital. The marriage, sadly, was an unhappy one, at least in part, one suspects due to the fact that each of the partners was devoted first and foremost to their work. In 1931, Florey became professor of pathology at Oxford University where his work on antimicrobial agents would inaugurate the antibiotic age. Enough penicillin was available by 1941 for clinical trials to begin: the results were spectacular. The deadly spectre of infection which had rendered even technically successful surgery a profoundly risky activity could be beaten.

In time Florey became president of the Royal Society and was awarded the Nobel Prize for physiology and medicine in 1945. He was knighted, appointed to the Légion d'Honneur and in 1965 was created Baron Florey of Adelaide and Marston, the year he was also appointed to the Order of Merit. He died in Oxford in 1968. Meanwhile, his wife, although struggling with deafness and chronic ill health, worked on at the BAH in a converted operating theatre, collaborating with her husband on the book *Antibiotics* and later publishing *The Clinical Application of Antibiotics* (London), in four volumes. She estimated that in the early trials of penicillin in Birmingham 1,000 working days were saved by giving penicillin to 35 patients.

Another pioneering woman who found a safe haven at the BAH was Olga Muller, a Polish Jew and Austrian by marriage. Escaping Nazi persecution, she and her husband and two daughters came to England in 1939. Her family, who remained in Poland, were sent to Auschwitz but survived. Her husband was interned as an enemy alien and her Austrian MD was not accepted in the United Kingdom. In desperate need of an income, Olga applied for a job as a nurse at the newly established Accident Hospital. When, after a few months her medical qualification was recognised, she became a part-time casualty officer, where she worked until the Austrian government eventually granted her a small pension, and she retired at the age of 81. Her sister and niece survived Auschwitz and later came to join her in Birmingham.

Douglas MacGilchrist Jackson arrived at the BAH in 1948. In 1953 he, like Essex-Lopresti, gave the prestigious Hunterian Lecture on the treatment of burns. As director of the Burns Unit he devised the "pin-prick" test which enables clinicians to differentiate partial thickness skin loss from full thickness skin loss within a few hours of admission to hospital (full thickness burns destroy nerves and the patient cannot feel them when they are touched, partial thickness burns leave nerves exposed to air and are intensely painful). Jackson was also an early advocate of "postage stamp grafts" and of treating more extensive deep burns by early tissue excision to the full depth of the burn followed by grafting. He produced important reports concerned with thermal injury affecting bones, joints and eyes.

In the final year of the War the pace of research activity meant that new laboratories for research and routine hospital work were needed and work began on them, utilising two wards and one of the three operating theatres.

The commitment of the hospital and its staff to the pioneering work of rehabilitation gathered pace as the War progressed and the need for industrial labour intensified. In 1942 a large gymnasium and additional rehabilitation, occupational and physiotherapy services were planned and opened the following year during which there were an astonishing 46,326 attendances, including 2,929 new patients. The hospital board alluded to the fact that *"each patient's rehabilitation needs are individual and are delivered by a variety of staff under the supervision of their surgeon".* Surprisingly, in 2023, this model of rehabilitation care is still not available to the majority of patients who need it.

On the prompting of Gissane, the BAH and the Austin Motor Company set up a workshop under the supervision of a works engineer. Medical supervision was provided by the works medical officer and Gissane, and all the men working in it were permanently or temporarily disabled. As soon as was possible during their rehabilitation training on industrial machinery began. Patients were paid a wage during their time in the workshop. In its first ten months, 150 men were returned either to their original job or to a job for which they had been retrained. In the last year of the War the rehabilitation service managed 5,380 new rehabilitation patients.

In order to further improve the service provided to the injured, in the early years of the War a short stay ward was opened to accommodate patients who needed admission for a simple procedure or a short period of recovery following a relatively minor injury. By 1944 over 2,000 patients each year were being admitted to it.

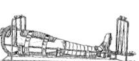

The care of the injured is not simply about medical and nursing care. As we shall see later, modern trauma care at its best requires an integrated team of specialists with a wide range of skills. The modern trauma team includes surgeons, intensive care specialists, physicians, microbiologists, occupational, physio- and speech therapists, social workers, psychologists and prosthetists. As we see the Accident Hospital developing through the War, the beginnings of such a multidisciplinary approach can be seen. At the time this was truly remarkable and reflected an unusual recognition by surgeons of the contributions of other professions and technicians in what was generally an extremely hierarchical organisation. In June 1943 a social services department was set up. The hospital board report states *"as will be realised from the forgoing...this hospital does not treat accidents but the people suffering from accidents.*

2. A Hospital at War

When the family wage earner breaks a limb, the problem goes far beyond the setting of a broken bone and the strengthening of the muscles for the accident has also caused a dislocation of the social, domestic and employment background of this citizen. The Social Service Department is that part of the Hospital treatment team which deals with this side of the accident problem."

That first year 1,552 inpatients were assisted and the service was subsequently extended to cover outpatients. The outpatients' department operated according to a model borrowed from industry. The doctor, nurses and secretaries stayed still and patients came past them: their dressings were removed, wounds inspected, treatment prescribed and dressings reapplied. The system was designed to see one patient every two minutes; a secretary sat next to the doctor ready to take notes regarding the examination and prepare a letter for the patient's general practitioner.

The Second World War brought problems as well as opportunities. There were inevitably staff shortages across all departments, especially clerical, maintenance and catering staff. In these pre-NHS days, the relationship between hospital managers and their staff was much closer than it is today. The hospital was run by a small committee, the management board, headed by the senior surgeon and matron, both steeped in clinical practice, expert in their fields and aware of the often-conflicting challenges of patient care and efficient management. A contemporary entry in the hospital board minutes notes *"the Board desires to express sympathy with senior officials who have to meet day-to-day problems without any stability of staff and indeed hardly daring to plan a day ahead."*

Despite these challenges, the hospital's commitment to improving the care of the injured through research and clinical development continued. In 1944 the department of physiology at Birmingham University was invited to study the quality of the diet fed to patients and staff. The hospital food was described as very satisfactory given wartime constraints on the availability of food.

In 1945 the trustees of the Bernhard Baron Charities Fund gave the sum of £5,000 (around £200,000 in contemporary values) for the development and maintenance of the Burns Unit which was renamed the Bernhard Baron Unit for the Treatment of Burns. Baron was born in Russia of French descent and made his fortune from inventing a machine which manufactured cigarettes with a paper cover, building his tobacco company into a multinational concern. A generous employer, he founded a superannuation fund for his workers, donated to hospitals and the Royal College of Surgeons and established retirement homes still run by his charity today. At the opening of a convalescent home in Brighton he remarked: *"I have nearly three thousand employees and I consider them my children, and anything I can do for them I will do. I have very faithful people and they all work with all their zeal to do the best they* can. There is only one happiness in life, and that is to protect others and to give to others." Perhaps it is no surprise that his charity gave so generously to the Birmingham Accident Hospital.

In 1943 Leonard Colebrook, an expert on the early antibacterial agent Prontosil moved, together with his burns team, from Glasgow Royal Infirmary to the BAH. One of those magisterial figures with a super-human capacity for work and total dedication to their profession so rarely seen today, Leonard Colebrook qualified at St Mary's Medical School in 1906, working on the treatment of tuberculosis and syphilis before the outbreak of war. Along with Sir Alexander Fleming he was a protégé of the great surgeon Sir Almroth Wright under whom he worked at the military hospital set up in a Boulogne casino during the Great War. As a consultant in London after the War, Colebrook was an early pioneer of antibiotics and his work on puerperal sepsis (an often-fatal infection contracted during childbirth) brought this scourge of women's lives to an end in this country. His work has been compared in importance to Lister's work on antisepsis. When war broke out again, although aged 56, Colebrook rejoined the Army as a bacteriologist where he introduced the dusting of wounds with the antibacterial sulphonilamide powder, which dramatically reduced the incidence of wound infections, sepsis and death. Later in the War he worked on burn treatment and it was as the founder of the BAH's Burns Unit that he came to Birmingham. He also contributed to a government-appointed war wounds sub-committee run by Sir Archibald McIndoe, founder of the famous "Guinea Pig Club" for badly burned servicemen. Throughout his career he had a particular determination to improve the lives of injured children and it was once said *"that Colebrook will never be thanked by those with most reason – the children who will not be listed in hospitals or Coroners reports"*.

Leonard Colebrook was known to his friends as "Coli" after the gut bacterium E.coli (one of his friends by the name of Porteous was known as "Proteus" after another bug). Colebrook was particularly impressed by the importance of airborne transfer of infection, and this work influenced the design of the BAH burns treatment room and more broadly many of the current ideas on the ventilation of surgical operating rooms. Colebrook retired in 1948 but continued to campaign for causes close to his heart. He received many awards from the medical and scientific community and was a fellow of the Royal Society, but curiously never received any national honour for his ground-breaking work. Colebrook's successor as head of the burns research laboratory, which became the MRC Industrial Injuries and Burns Research Unit in 1952, was Edward Lowbury.

Perhaps inevitably, Colebrook became a pioneer fire safety campaigner. His campaigning against the risks unguarded fires posed to children and the dangers of cheap flammable nightclothes would lead to the *Heating Appliances and Fireguards Act 1952* which made it illegal to sell a new gas, electric or oil heater which was not fitted with an adequate guard. The hospital's annual reports had drawn attention to the frequency with which children's nightgowns caught fire as early as 1945, recommending that fireguards be better designed, and that children's clothes should not be made of highly flammable materials.

Every modern hospital has a clinical photography department which produces images for teaching, to monitor treatment, to illustrate patient information literature and for publication. Such a department was opened at the BAH in 1942, when it acquired the extra job of photographing for storage the huge quantities of radiographic images which were accumulating as the hospital became increasingly busy. Other early and ground-breaking projects included photographing bacteriological specimens as slides making then easier to interpret and documenting skin lesions for the MRC Industrial Injuries Research Unit. By 1947 the department was taking almost 11,000 images a year!

As the hospital developed and its workload grew, its relationship with money remained a challenge and it continued in those pre-NHS days to rely heavily on local support from individuals and industry. Early providers of funding, apart from the City of Birmingham and the Department of Health, would include the Birmingham Hospitals Contribution Association, ICI Metals, the Austin Motor Company, W&T Avery (Birmingham manufacturers of weighing scales since 1730), Cadbury's and Guest, Keen and Nettlefold (GKN).

The radical and farsighted decision to open the Birmingham Accident Hospital and Rehabilitation Centre was surely vindicated when, in 1944 in the House of Commons, Sir Patrick Hannon said of the BAH: "*The hospital is giving the lead in the rehabilitation and restoration of injured and wounded men to make them fit for industry, and their work should be known throughout the length and breadth of the land. It is a particularly ambitious venture, which has received substantial support and the success of its experiment has been remarkable. What has happened is that the Accident Hospital, under admirable control and direction, is in contact with various works, and as the process of restoration to working capacity goes on in the hospital the men are gradually brought back in context with the work in which they engaged in the particular factory before the injury. Even before full capacity is reached, they may be back at work and his work may go side by side with the work of restoration.*"

As a mark of the national esteem in which the hospital was held, and possibly also of its work through the War years, Their Majesties King George VI and Queen Elizabeth honoured the hospital with a visit on the 7th November 1945.

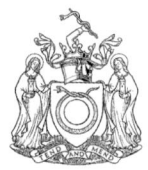

First Interlude

The Birth of Orthopaedics

IN THE CORNER of the graveyard of Otley's Parish Church of All Saints in Yorkshire's West Riding, stands an unusual memorial: a miniature copy of the entrance to the nearby Bramhope Tunnel, erected as a memorial to all the "navvies" who lost their lives during the tunnel's construction. Unsurprisingly, the early Victorians were not known for their safety culture and the transformation of the early

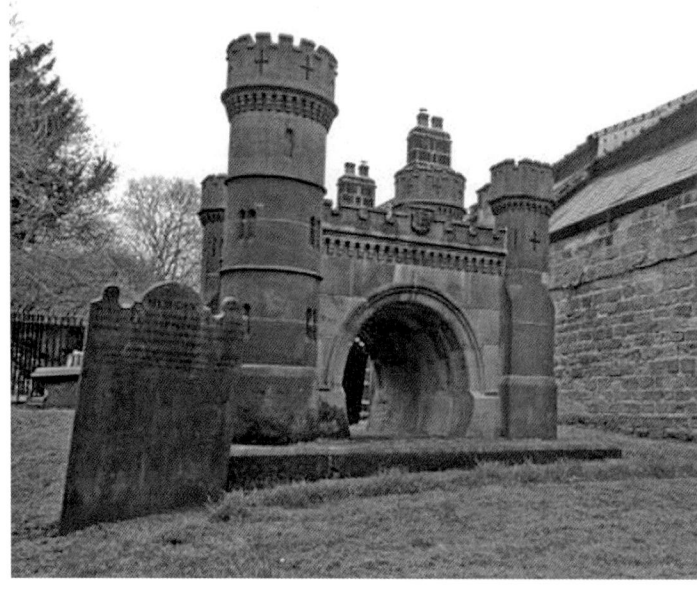

Otley's Bramhope Tunnel Memorial.

and mid-nineteenth century was indeed built on the bodies of the itinerant workmen and labourers who toiled to make Britain the World's first industrial nation. Life at the forefront of the Industrial Revolution was a hazardous business as men, materials and processes were tested to their limit, driven by capitalism at its most free range.

Aside from Huskisson, whom we have already met falling under a train, lives were lost to exploding boilers, roof and bridge collapses, explosions, toxic chemical processes and the rapid and uncontrolled mechanisation of what were once cottage industries. The Victorians also succumbed to mercury poisoning (hat makers – hence the expression "mad as a hatter"), phosphorus vapour (matchstick makers), arsenic (cosmetics, dyes and wallpaper), scrotal cancer (chimney sweeps), cotton fibres (weavers) and coal dust, amongst many other noxious agents. Inevitably the industrial poor bore the brunt of this trauma, their ability to survive it compromised by exhaustion, poor diet, insanitary housing, little or no education and rampant infectious disease in the absence of any formal structure of health care. Equally inevitably, the clinicians of the BAH would eventually be interested in the whole spectrum of industrial disease and its prevention.

The Industrial Revolution and the massive industrial expansion that followed began in the mid-eighteenth century and transformed the landscape of Britain and the working lives of the majority of its people. Cities expanded massively and working lives became regimented and coordinated to achieve maximum manufacturing output, often at a devastating cost in lives lost or blighted. We have seen the growth of Birmingham; between the early eighteenth century and the end of the nineteenth, the population of Manchester grew from 10,000 to 2.3 million and of Leeds from 16,000 to 160,000, a level of growth mirrored by all the industrial and manufacturing cities of the United Kingdom. The main areas of industrial growth were textiles, heavy engineering, industrial innovation and iron and steel manufacture. There were, inevitably, regional variations; the North West and South Yorkshire were associated with textile manufacture, with Manchester earning the nickname *Cottonopolis*.

The Midlands offered a more varied industrial landscape, although one largely based on metal working. Birmingham manufactories made nails, screws, nuts and bolts and other small items such as pen nibs. Joseph Chamberlain, Mayor of Birmingham, pioneer of civic development and foreign secretary, never seen without an orchid from his Moseley glasshouses in his buttonhole, made his fortune in screw manufacturing. Other industries included glass making, armaments manufacture (north-bound train travellers, from the city centre still pass the Birmingham Proof House established by act of Parliament in 1813, at the request and the expense of the Birmingham Gun Trade, to provide a testing facility for firearms) and the making of jewellery. Cars and chocolate would follow. The Black Country to the North and

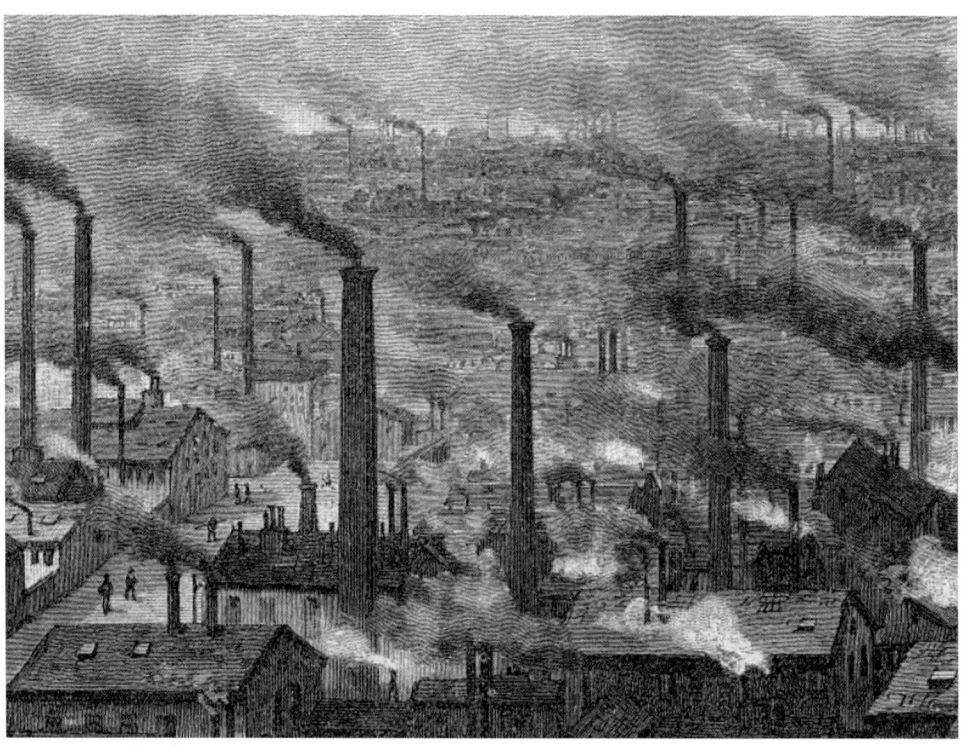

The industrial city.

West of Birmingham would be associated with coal mining, iron and steel production, glass making and brick works.

Working hours were long (12 to 16 hours a day, six days a week), conditions poor and employees, including children, at least initially, were unprotected by health and safety legislation. In some areas, enlightened employers would offer what was effectively a private welfare state for their staff, although of a more paternalistic and restrictive kind than would now be accepted. These enlightened employers, of which the most well-known is probably Sir Titus Salt of Saltaire, West Yorkshire, were rare. Mechanisation needed unskilled employees and pay was consequently low. Skilled craftsmen and women carrying out piecework from their own homes almost entirely passed into memory. The massive increase in housing in Britain's cities led to poor living as well as working conditions, infectious diseases were rife and social support almost non-existent. Many of Birmingham's urban poor lived in tightly packed squalid back-to-back houses which sometimes also contained small workshops. Once a common feature of Birmingham's cityscape, the handful which survive now belong to the National Trust and are open as a tourist attraction.

First Interlude

Workers were generally in poor physical shape, unhealthy and chronically tired. Machinery was unfenced and factories were poorly lit; unsurprisingly, accidents were common. Medical care was limited, being provided by charity hospitals. Any injury which resulted in an inability to work inevitably led to unemployment, increased poverty, potential starvation, homelessness and the workhouse. The first legislation designed to improve safety in the Victorian workplace did not appear until 1844 when the Factories Act was passed by Parliament. The Act made the inspecting of industrial premises and the reporting of accidents compulsory.

More surprisingly, there was no medical specialty dedicated to the care of the injured. Because most of those injured were poor and unable to pay for treatment, their management inevitably occurred in the charity hospitals where care was provided for free. Surgery for internal injuries was in its infancy and operations for internal bleeding were rarely performed and even more rarely successful.

Although the term orthopaedics, from the Greek ὀρθός *orthos* (correct) and παιδίον *paidion* (child), was coined in 1741 by the French physician Nicholas Andry, its emphasis was far from the management of trauma and no speciality existed within the medical profession; the management of fractures and dislocations was beneath the notice of university educated practitioners and remained the domain of unqualified, although often highly effective bone setters.

The greatest bone setter of them all was the buccaneering Hugh Owen Thomas, a man who was simultaneously the last of the freebooting bone setters and, as a conventionally qualified doctor, the father of British orthopaedic surgery. Much remains mysterious about Thomas, although his greatest invention transformed the survival rates of injured servicemen in World War I. He was the descendant of a child shipwrecked on the shores on Anglesey in 1745 and who adopted the name of the family that took him in. Young Evan Thomas became a bone setter, a career followed by his descendants into the twentieth century. Evan's grandson established himself in practice in Liverpool where, unqualified, he was repeatedly taken to court by medical practitioners who challenged his entitlement to practice. A professional lifetime of challenge and jealousy during which his house was at one stage burnt down caused him to compel all his five sons to attend medical school. Thus his son Hugh Owen was both the latest in a line of bone setters and a qualified doctor; ideally positioned to establish the speciality of orthopaedics and transform the lives of the injured. Despite this, there is no doubt that he was an awkward fit in the nineteenth century medical profession. His appearance was unusual, a little over five feet tall, he

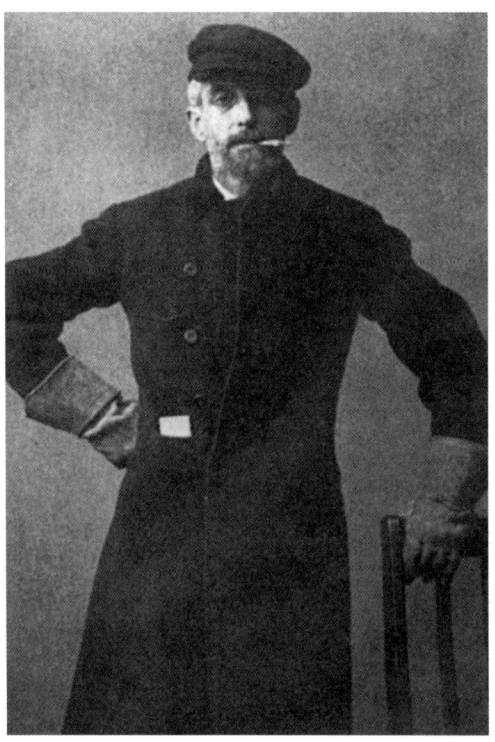

Hugh Owen Thomas, the Cripples' Champion.

invariably wore a long coat buttoned to the chin combined with a cap at a jaunty angle. A cigarette always dangled from his lips and the overall effect was of a medical Dick Dastardly. His temperament was difficult and his quarrels frequent; he was said by fellow doctors, who generally loathed him, to have broken clients' bones so as to be able to charge to fix them. Given his reputation for compassion for the poor, amongst whom he established his practice, this is almost certainly a slur spread by his professional enemies.

After studying in Edinburgh and London Hugh worked with his father before characteristically falling out with him and setting up practice in one of the poorer areas of Liverpool where he worked in private practice six days a week and gave his services free of charge to the poor on Sundays. Amongst the city's poor he became known as the Cripples' Champion. Aside from his work amongst Liverpool's working classes, this unlikely pioneer transformed the management of injuries and the diseases of bones. Given his family history, his decision to specialise in the injuries and diseases of the locomotor system was probably inevitable and he was particularly interested in the scourge of bone tuberculosis, then a common cause of illness, disability and death amongst rich and poor alike. He was an early advocate of rest which was to be *"enforced that the patient's ordinary movements will not materially jar the joint, uninterrupted, even momentarily, so as not to arrest or delay the progress to cure, and prolonged to secure beyond relapse the resolution of the disease"*. He created the splint which still bears his name, as well as other splints to encourage immobilization. He also invented multiple instruments for the management of fractures. Owen Thomas was the uncle of Sir Robert Jones, arguably the greatest of British orthopaedic surgeons, of whom we shall hear more a little later.

First Interlude

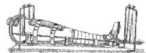

It is unsurprising, but little acknowledged that it was the Victorians who first recognised that society had a responsibility to its members and that unfettered commercialism must be constrained for the public good. It was the Victorians too who began to put the necessary structures in place through legislation, including the Factory Act of 1833, which restricted the working day in textile mills to 12 hours for 13 to 17 year olds and eight hours for those aged between 9 and 12. The subsequent 1844 Factories Act was in many ways the first health and safety legislation, requiring that all dangerous machinery was to be securely fenced off, and making failure to do so a criminal offence. Further acts would follow in 1847, 1878, 1891 and 1895. Nevertheless, the workplace remained a dangerous environment and the injured had little to fall back on in terms of treatment or social support.

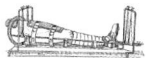

In 2002, Isambard Kingdom Brunel was second only to Sir Winston Churchill in the BBC's Greatest Briton competition. The engineer of the Great Western Railway, SS *Great Britain*, the Clifton Suspension Bridge and numerous other projects was without doubt an engineering pioneer of towering genius; he was also an obsessive who drove his schemes without much regard for safety or workers' welfare, and of whom it might well be said that many of his projects were doomed to failure by their own grandiosity. It is Brunel's exact contemporary and fellow engineer Thomas Brassey who concerns us here, and the contrasts between the two are striking. Brassey was one of those Victorian titans of industry whose work and achievements are almost impossible to comprehend 150 years later. Born the son of a farmer in 1805 (Brunel was born the following year), at the age of 16 he was apprenticed as a civil engineer working on the new road from Shrewsbury to Holyhead where he came to the notice of the great Thomas Telford, builder of the suspension bridge across the Menai Straits to Anglesey and the ferry to Ireland. Entering into business on his own account at the age of 21, from the start his work was characterised by innovation in materials transport, logistics and management. From his first contract for four miles of road, his success was built on sound organisation, innovation and what we would now call "man-management skills". He became a leading contractor in building Britain's new railway network, ultimately constructing around one third of the track laid down in the nineteenth century. By the time he died in 1870, he had built one mile in every 20 of the World's railways. His interests were astonishing, and matched only by his capacity for hard work. He built railways in Canada, Australia, India and South America as well as docks, railway buildings, bridges, tunnels, steamships, mines, locomotives, sewers, and marine telegraphy. He was also a shareholder in Brunel's SS *Great Eastern* which is where the paths of these two great Victorians cross. At the height of his powers he had wanted to build a tunnel under the English Channel, but this never came to fruition. If it had, there is little doubt that it would have been completed under budget and on time. On his death he left a fortune equivalent to £600 million in today's money.

Most remarkably for a man of such achievements, nobody had a bad word to say about Brassey, who was widely admired by peers and employees alike. When the Barentin Viaduct which he was building with local lime as stipulated in the contract, collapsed in 1846, Brassey rebuilt it at his own expense. His military railway built to aid beleaguered British forces during the Crimean War was constructed at cost price. When the conventional vision of a Victorian tycoon was of a Gradgrind or a Melmotte, Brassey set new standards, providing libraries and reading rooms for his employees. His navvies were not itinerant labourers, but rather a *"highly skilled mobile army"* who were cared for and received a generous wage, clothing and shelter, as well as financial support in difficult times.

Importantly for our story, Brassey passed his pioneering approach to employment on to his protégé Thomas Walker, who first worked alongside him on the Canadian Grand Trunk Railway in 1852. Walker (1828-1889) was the civil engineering contractor responsible for, amongst other projects, the Severn Tunnel, the London District Railway and, his final project, the Manchester Ship Canal. The ship canal connecting the Irish Sea with Manchester was the greatest engineering challenge of the nineteenth century: its 36 miles took six years to build and required, apart from the canal itself, the construction of multiple locks, bridges, weirs, a swing bridge and a canal-carrying aqueduct capable of swinging out of the way to allow large ships to pass. An average of 12,000 workers were employed during the canal's creation, with a peak of 17,000. Navvies were paid four pence ha'penny per hour for a ten hour day, 200 miles of temporary railway track, 180 locomotives, more than 6,000 trucks and wagons as well as more than 300 pieces of steam driven equipment, not including 100 steam excavators, were used. Most importantly for our story, however, was the fact that, like his mentor, Brassey, Walker provided excellent facilities for his employees including meeting halls, recreational facilities and accommodation. He also provided hospital facilities. In fact, the Manchester Ship Canal building project saw the establishment of the World's first comprehensive service for the injured and the doctor in charge of it, was a young Robert Jones, the founder of modern orthopaedics and the nephew of Hugh Owen Thomas. Under Jones' system casualties were taken by rail to the nearest of three hospitals each

First Interlude

with 20 beds and a resident surgeon. Medical facilities capable of dealing with serious injuries were distributed at intervals along the 36 miles of canal.

Sir Robert Jones, 1st Baronet, (1857-1933) was born in Llandudno, North Wales but brought up in London where his father attempted, largely unsuccessfully, to earn a living as a writer. Aged 16 he went to live with his uncle, Hugh Owen Thomas in Liverpool, where he gained an education in fracture management and splintage. Qualifying from Liverpool Medical School in 1878, Jones worked with his uncle, developing the fledgling speciality of modern orthopaedic surgery. In 1888 he was appointed a surgeon-superintendent of the Manchester Ship Canal. During the construction of the canal, Jones personally managed 3,000 cases and performed 300 operations; inevitably standards were set for the development of a new speciality. In 1894, Jones and a colleague founded the British Orthopaedic Society, although most surgeons operating on trauma cases were still general surgeons and the society folded after four years. Like Dr John Hall Edwards, Jones was a pioneer of X-rays in medicine. In 1896, the same year as Hall Edwards' pioneering studies, Jones took an X-ray of a boy's wrist to identify the location of a bullet. The exposure took two hours and the case became the first published account of the medical use of X-rays. Unlike Hall Edwards, Jones did not subsequently dedicate his career to the medical use of imaging.

When the Great War broke out in 1914, Robert Jones was mobilised in the Royal Army Medical Corps. It rapidly became clear to him that the management of the fractures common in industrialised warfare was far from adequate and his relentless campaigning led to the establishment of military orthopaedic hospitals. Subsequently appointed Inspector of Military Orthopaedics, at one point he was responsible for more than 30,000 beds on the continent and at home. His London hospital in Hammersmith became the exemplar for both British and American military orthopaedic hospitals. His most lasting achievement and the one with which he will forever be associated, however, was the introduction of the Thomas splint for the initial treatment of fractures of the femur which dramatically reduced the mortality of this previously fatal injury. The importance of war-time experience in trauma management will be a theme to which we return.

By the end of the War, Jones was a major general. He was knighted in 1917, awarded a

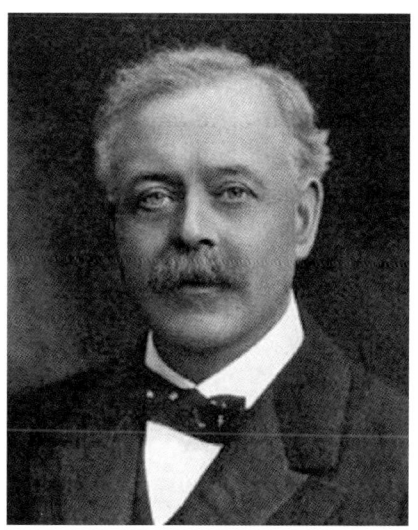

Sir Robert Jones Bt.

The "Acci"

KBE and a CB in 1919 and became a baronet in 1920. Honoured by the USA, and the recipient of multiple honorary degrees, he died in 1933 and is buried in Liverpool's Anglican Cathedral. More important than his personal honours was the fact that he paid a unique role in establishing orthopaedics and the specialist treatment of the injured as part of conventional medical practice, a role recognised when he was made first president of the Institute of Orthopaedic Surgery. A specialist hospital in Oswestry still bears his name and fittingly, as we shall see, a statue of Sir Robert was unveiled by the Duke of Cambridge in the Defence Medical Services new rehabilitation centre at Stanford Hall in 2018.

Orthopaedics was on the map and the torch would be carried by the specialists at the Birmingham Accident Hospital and Rehabilitation centre.

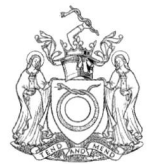

Chapter 3

A Hospital at Work and at Play

AS LATE AS the 1980s, British hospitals were strikingly different from the huge teaching hospitals of today. They were more than places of work; they were small inward-looking communities under the gimlet eye of matron (think Hattie Jacques, but slimmer and considerably less amorous) and fiercely proud of their reputations. Not only was the hospital a place of work, but for the junior doctors and junior nursing staff it was home too.

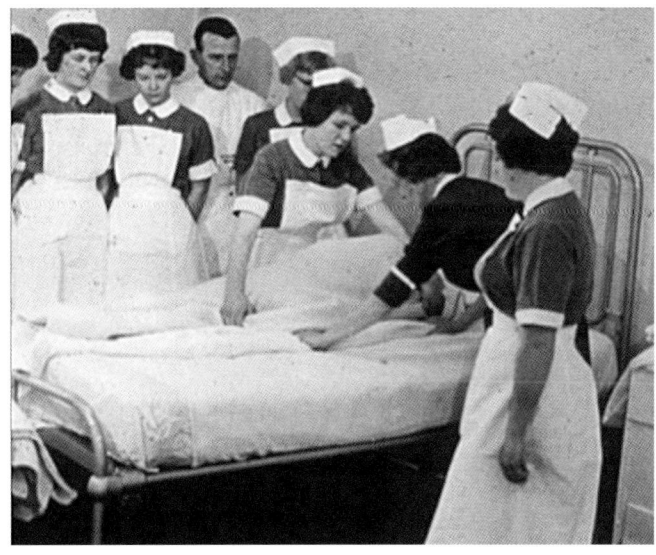

"And then we roll the patient onto their side, Sister".

The term junior doctor is a strange one, including as it does all hospital doctors who are not yet consultants. It is a term that seems now to cause offence, 30 years ago it was simply accepted as meaning "not a consultant". Until the twenty-first century, when consultants started to be appointed at a younger age, these doctors could be anything from their early 20s, to 40: they were the backbone of a service which would be unrecognisable to today's NHS staff. The level of responsibility expected of junior doctors was startling. In 1947 there was consternation at a BAH medical staff meeting when one of the hospital's anaesthetists opposed a surgical proposal that the housemen (the most junior doctors of all, newly qualified) should administer the anaesthetics for trauma surgery.

Until changes brought about by the European Working Time Directive and in response to changes in medical education, the foundation of clinical care was the team led by the consultant (with shades of Sir Lancelot Spratt – "*Pursue me, pursue me...*"). Below the consultant was the senior registrar who could generally do anything the consultant could do and whose main task was to make sure that the consultant spent as little time in the hospital out of hours as possible, only being called in when his skills and experience were needed. To a degree, this was a necessary protection as consultants worked very heavy rotas throughout their careers. The senior registrar, like the consultant wore a suit. Next in the pecking order was the registrar, who was considered rather grand by those below him and sported a jacket when on ward rounds. Registrars with pretensions, usually of the surgical variety, were occasionally seen in a suit, to general derision from their junior colleagues. At the bottom of the pile, apart from medical students, obviously, were the senior house officers and house officers, or housemen; women were still unusual amongst the medical staff. White coats were the mark of junior medical staff, their pockets full in inverse proportion to their seniority. Hierarchies were observed: seniors were addressed by their title – especially surgeons, who were most particular about being "Mr" rather than "Dr". At the BAH medical staff wore white coats with red labels indicating their status, until the hospital closed. Being thrown a consultant's keys and asked to bring their car to the main entrance was one of the tasks allotted to juniors who, generally, recognised the experience of their seniors and were happy to oblige.

The junior doctor's next job was usually awarded on the personal recommendation of their current supervising consultant. Candidates who could not count on a phone call from their consultant to the chair of the appointment committee the night before the interviews were unlikely to be successful in their applications.

The first two years of medical training at Birmingham Medical School were, visits to the BAH aside, entirely non-clinical. Patients were not encountered until the third year. Much of the second year was spent in the dissecting room where hours were spent acquiring a minute knowledge of anatomy. Each group of students worked on the same body throughout the year. Gloves were not worn and a faint miasma of the dissecting room followed students around. Clinically, medical students at Birmingham Medical School had the privilege of access to patients from Worcester to Coventry, Stoke-on-Trent to Warwick. The clinical exposure was remarkable and the training took the form of an apprenticeship under the supervision of consultants in the necessary specialties. Academic education was left to the student's own initiative, subject only to passing the regular examinations. Clinical procedures, often quite invasive, were learned by "watching one", then "doing one", traditionally followed by "teaching one". Junior medical students attached to surgical firms were known as dressers after their Victorian role in dressing the wounds of post-operative patients, and on medical firms as clerks as it was their responsibility to "clerk" the patients, that is to take a history and perform an examination before completing the patient's notes. Consultants expected their students to "present" the patients, giving a brief history and summary of the examination findings as well as the test results, which they were expected to know and were not permitted to write down. Blood results too had to be learned, or written on the palm of the hand or just guessed. The ability to estimate the patient's blood count based on how pale they were was a useful skill. Ward rounds were frequently interrupted for tea and biscuits with sister and followed by an informal meeting in the consultants' dining room where ideas were shared. Now seen as a mark of hierarchy, doctors' dining rooms often provided an opportunity for sorting out tricky clinical issues in confidence or supporting stressed and exhausted juniors. Ward rounds on a Saturday morning were routine and sometimes appeared more of a test of surgical machismo than an exercise of value to the patients.

Out of hours, the hospital was the preserve of the juniors whose life revolved around the doctors' mess where they lived and for whom the hospital was both place of work and home. Breakfast was taken communally when on-call bleeps were handed over to the next on-call team and sick patients could be discussed. Evenings were spent in the hospital doctors' bar or social club or revising for professional examinations. As late as the 1980s, one Birmingham pub popular with doctors from the hospital across the road had a hospital telephone extension in the bar. The BAH canteen served free food for night staff well into the 1980s and medical students were encouraged to stay overnight in an empty bed! Amorous opportunities for junior doctors occurred almost entirely with nurses with the occasional physiotherapist or pharmacist. Even now a whole generation of doctors remain married to members of one the few groups they came into contact with as part of a life that was entirely hospital focussed. In most hospitals switchboard operators with their finger on the social pulse knew which room in the nurses' home they needed to ring in order to put calls through to errant junior doctors. Marriage before reaching the heights of registrar was unusual. Medical students from Birmingham University attended the BAH from their first year, learning the basics of wound management by apprenticeship. Students were on call when the team to which they were attached was on call. During training in specialties such as obstetrics, the nights were split between the available students so working every other night was far from uncommon. Academic work was completed in the nights off. In some hospitals junior doctors were expected not only to live in, but to ask permission from their consultant when they wanted a night off.

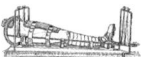

By the end of the Second World War, the structure that would be retained until closure was established: three clinical teams (unimaginatively called team one, team two and team three) each consisting of two consultants and the requisite assortment of junior staff. Each consultant was on duty every sixth night and all the consultants either lived in the hospital when they were on call or within a few minutes' drive of it. The Accident Hospital consultants expected to be, and were, called in on a regular basis. When a consultant was on call, the entire team were present, but at all times, a member of each team was available within the hospital to look after their own inpatients from previous nights on call (or "take" as it was often called). There was therefore always a doctor in the hospital who knew every patient, a degree of continuity now long lost. As a result, the juniors did what was referred to as a "1 in 3". Hours outside the "normal working day" were paid at one third of the normal rate. Weekends started at 08.00 on Friday and finished around 17.00 on Monday and sleep was a bonus. Until the relatively recent development of the role of the nurse, tasks such as the administration of antibiotics, catheterisation and the passing of assorted tubes fell to the junior medical staff. Behaviour on the wards could on occasion be raucous and included trolley races and water fights with bladder syringes. Hospital corridors were ideally suited to golf practice and on at least one occasion a car was driven into the Queen Elizabeth Hospital entrance hall.

Consultant behaviour varied from the malign to the genuinely caring. The consultants who were most respected, and whose jobs were the most sought after, were those whose respect had to be earned; once earned they were potentially allies for life. Many a distinguished career was built on the foundations of striving to demonstrate high standards and commitment to a demanding "boss". Most were aware of the challenges of life as a junior doctor and at least tried not to make them any more difficult. Some had a reputation for never being available and treating their juniors with disinterest or disdain. A notable British Medical Journal of the time reported that one deceased consultant *"taught by humiliation"*. Being made to feel small for failing to present a patient to the consultant's satisfaction was, whatever the educationalists might say, a singularly effective way of ensuring that the beleaguered student never repeated the experience. Most consultants took their clinical role and teaching responsibilities with great seriousness and many were capable of remarkable kindness to their beleaguered junior staff, demonstrated by such acts as lending a new junior doctor a month's salary when the hospital failed to pay them. Most were more impressed by hard work than brilliance, some were extraordinarily funny, some were capable of inspiring remarkable affection and loyalty amongst their staff. In the right hands, ward rounds were therapeutic, educational and entertaining in equal measure. Few were dull. Bad behaviour which would result in disciplinary action today was then almost admired. It was rumoured that a very senior physician had never, in a 30 year career of examining for a particular Royal College, actually passed anyone. Needless to say, this was considered only to add to the kudos of those who did manage to pass (presumably thanks to other examiners).

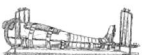

The nursing staff formed a similarly tight-knit community based around the wards and the nurses' home. Matron ruled the hospital with a rod of iron and the ward sisters ruled the wards, the patients and visiting medical staff in a similar manner. In many hospitals sister was known by the name of her ward. Sister would greet the consultant at the beginning of his round and accompany him during it, retiring at the end to her office for tea. Medical students asked her permission to visit patients on the ward. Qualified nurses wore starched hats, student nurses wore paper ones marked with a blue stripe for each year of their training. Brand new student nurses had a red stripe on their hats, the significance of which was subject to a degree of scurrilous as well as innocent speculation. Nurses in training lived in the nurses' home which was, in theory at least, run along the lines of a strict girls' boarding school.

The annual social high spot was the hospital Christmas show, a scatological and suggestive review featuring much cross-dressing and near-nudity which held up the consultants and others in authority to ridicule. On one memorable occasion, whenever a particular consultant was mentioned, a "full" bedpan was carried across the stage. Equally, on the other hand, the most approachable consultants might be invited to take part, a considerable social accolade amongst the consultant body. All the proceeds were donated to charity and the show was truly a hospital effort. In one Birmingham hospital the sewing room produced a complete set of tutus for the largest and hairiest (male) doctors to perform Swan Lake. This was a hard drinking, hard playing culture, but one in which medicine was seen as a way of life rather than simply an occupation. Inevitably, *The Acci* presented a show by the "Bath Row Amateur *Traumatic* Society".

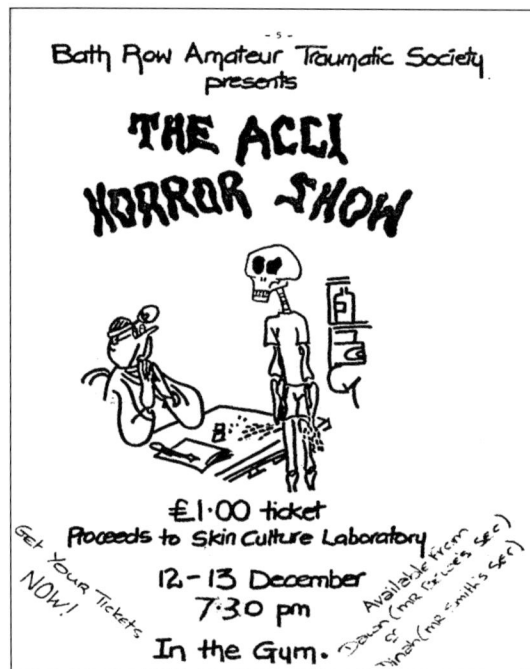

An "Amateur Traumatic Society" poster.

The Accident Hospital had an active social club from soon after its opening until its closure. A letter to the editor of the hospital magazine reads:

To Socialize or Not?
Who wants a social club? I do, and I know lots more who do too. In a hospital with this amount [sic] of staff why is it that nobody seems to have the enthusiasm to get a club going?

There's an idea going around that if we could find a room somewhere in the hospital where we could let rip – (so to speak!) there would be plenty of willing, enthusiastic helpers to get the room transformed into a place with a bit of atmosphere – it needn't cost much either. Tables and chairs could be made out of crates, a few soft lights around and it would be great.

It could be somewhere to go during lunch hour or for staff staying late at night – just to have a cup of coffee and mingle with others, instead of staying "departmentalized" with only the steam bugs for company.

I expect someone will find fault though with any idea put forward which could mean a bit of fun. But please give it a thought this time, Mr. Editor.

Lonely, of B.A.H

3. A Hospital at Work and at Play

Naturally, the club had a licence from the local justices to sell alcohol and a bar and lounge area were created, mainly by the efforts of a few amateur DIY experts. The old bar became the home for disco equipment when additional rooms were made available. The club was staffed by a married couple and opened at lunchtime when it served light meals and in the evenings, when it provided a bolt hole for junior doctors from the "Crows' Nest", as the medical staff accommodation was called, and the nurses' home. Serendipitously, the club was sponsored by the next-door Davenport's Brewery. For those on call, there was a "half-pint rule" and for those on the late shift which finished at 21.30 it was a useful rendezvous. Unsurprisingly, as the central point of a community of largely young people, a wide range of cups and trophies were available for various sporting activities.

The hospital community did not only include the staff, patients were a vital part of it too. Both staff and patients contributed to the hospital magazine which was on occasion forthright in its criticism of managerial policy.

The annual hospital ball was a highlight of the hospital year and an opportunity for consultants, nurses and juniors to let their hair down on an equal footing. Each year there was a nurses' Christmas dinner, consultant staff Christmas dinner and ancillary staff Christmas dinner. The consultants, together with their less enthusiastic families, were expected to attend the hospital on Christmas day to carve the turkey

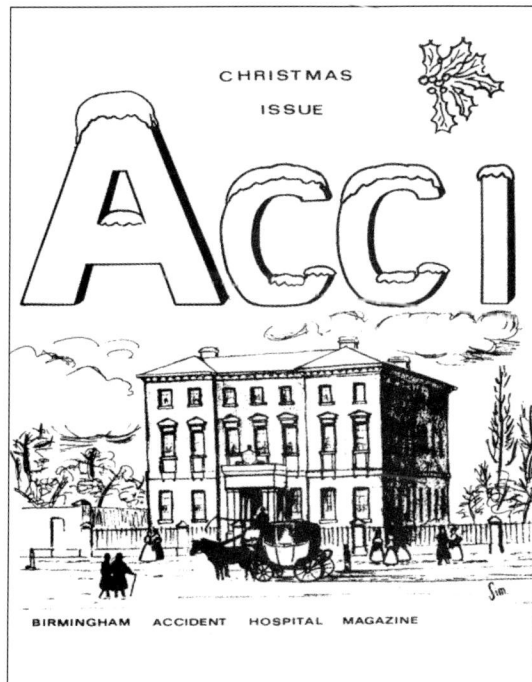

The Accident Hospital Magazine.

and distribute the patients' food whilst the junior medical staff indulged in a Christmas toast with the nursing staff on each ward in turn. Each night of the year, the surgical team on call would eat together with members of the team often taking it in turn to cook or calling on the services of one of the city's many takeaways.

It is a mark of the closeness and strength of the Accident Hospital community, and of the fact that hospitals played a much greater part in the lives of those who worked in them 50 years ago than they do now, that staff reunions began almost as soon as the hospital closed its doors and continue to this day. These reunions have often been connected with charitable fundraising as well as providing an opportunity to meet old friends and colleagues. But above all, there is a sense of pride: as the former Prime Minister Harold Macmillan once put it, *"it is a great thing at some time in your life to be associated with something which is quite first class"*. The reunions are held in hotels or private homes, on one occasion that of Geraldine Amos, founder of Birmingham's Home from Hospital Charity which still provides support to patients returning to their own homes; one of the former consultants is usually prevailed upon to give a speech.

Birmingham Accident Hospital Medical Society was established shortly after the War in order to promote academic development and encourage innovation in patient management. The society met almost every week and was attended by medical staff and invited guests. Each year began with a presidential address from Professor Gissane and the election of the year's chairman and secretary. Expert speakers from outside the hospital and from abroad attended and regular research updates were offered. Complex cases were discussed and the cases of patients who had died were reviewed in detail. These activities prefigured by decades the multidisciplinary case reviews and mortality and morbidity (M&M) meetings of modern trauma care.

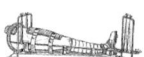

The Accident Hospital undoubtedly had more than its fair share of royal and distinguished visitors. Some of these came in the wake of the hospital's response to the Pub Bombings and we shall return to these later. Of the others, the most celebrated was that of Princess Diana who came to reopen the Children's Burns Unit. On her arrival, a bouquet was presented by a little girl who had been treated for severe burns. Characteristically, Princess Diana took the girl by the hand and asked if she would like to join her for the visit, which she was only too excited to do. In 1988 after her visit, Princess Michael of Kent wrote thanking the hospital's staff: *"It was important for me because I wanted anyway to have the chance of talking to you and your staff, and of course the patients about the steps we can take to reduce road accidents. I learned much that would have otherwise been less easily revealed, which was most useful. But the thing I*

3. A Hospital at Work and at Play

valued above all was the tremendous professionalism and high morale shown by everyone in the hospital, which was greatly infectious. I was so impressed, and clearly the accident victims could not find themselves in better hands".

As we have seen, from its foundation as the Queen's Hospital, what would become the Accident Hospital had very deep roots in its community. The flourishing league of friends which supported the hospital over many years was a manifestation of this. The league raised funds for equipment, provided volunteers for the hospital and sought to raise its profile. Volunteers provided tea on the wards and general assistance to patients and staff alike. The *Ladies Linen League*, founded by Mrs Gissane, made garments and comforts for patients, not to mention costumes for the Christmas show. Amongst the genteel activities organised were sherry evenings (with cheese and pineapple on sticks!), coffee mornings, whist drives and hospital bazaars – often referred to in those days as "sales of work". Much money was raised by street collections in the city centre. In later years, members of the league paid an annual subscription of 5/- (25p). An appeal was run in conjunction with the *Birmingham Mail* and in the early days at least, links with local industry were strong, with employers seeing the hospital, at least in part, as a means of returning their employees to work as soon as possible.

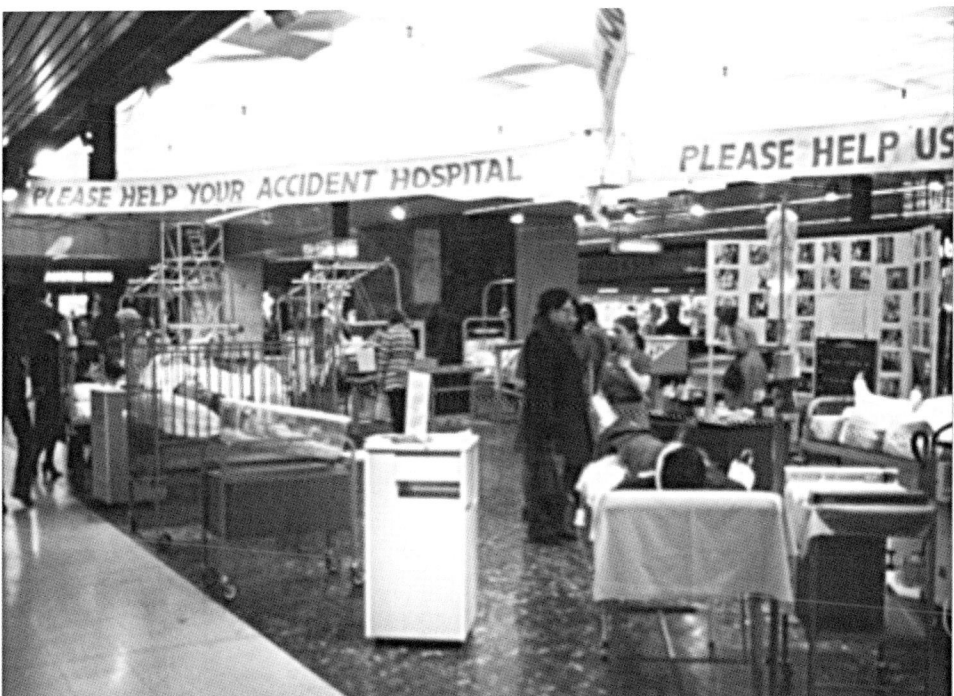

City centre fundraising.

Hospital wards, too, were different from those occupied by today's patients. The majority were "Nightingale" wards with a long row of beds down each side and a nurses' table lit by a single bulb in the middle. Although much more formal in terms of behaviour, considerable attention was given to making the patients feel at home, and generally longer stays than usual today made this more important. Each ward had a day room meaning that patients were not compelled through lack of any alternative to lie in bed or sit in a chair next to their bed. The day room was often wreathed in cigarette smoke but offered the opportunity for some communal television watching (three channels only) and board games. A budgerigar in a cage was often found in one corner. Most patients' bedside tables were loaded with cards and flowers, an encouragement to recovery, but a challenge to those whose tables were bare. A trolley selling newspapers, sweets and toiletries visited each ward daily. At Christmas, as we have seen, the consultant, his wife and family attended the highly decorated ward to carve the turkey supplied whole by the hospital kitchens with all the trimmings. A wide variety of alcohol was available and consumed by patients and staff alike, all of whom felt they were part of something a little larger than a system built on statistics, targets and arbitrary measures of efficiency.

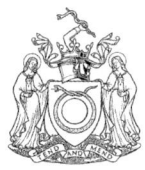

Chapter 4

State of the Art

IMMEDIATELY AFTER THE War, the hospital was in a poor state of repair and its staff, like the nation itself, were exhausted. Nevertheless, the foundations had been laid, and the necessary experience gained, for the achievement of more than 30 years of ground-breaking patient care and research activity. In the second half of the 1940s, a series of great names of trauma medicine, including Ruscoe Clarke, Edward Lowbury and Leonard Colebrook, would join the Accident Hospital team, bringing with them extensive wartime experience of military wounds and their treatment, which was of immense benefit in driving forward civilian trauma care. The transfer of skills learned in wartime practice would inform civilian medicine and surgery and lead to dramatic improvements. As we shall see, this transfer of military surgical skills and experience would again, during the wars in Iraq and Afghanistan, lead to the greatest advances in trauma care since the immediate post-Second World War period and once more Birmingham clinicians would play an essential role.

The rota was based on a three-week cycle and 24 hour days on "take" or 80-hour weekends. On a three-week cycle, this resulted in seven 24 hour periods on resident duty for all the housemen and women, senior house officers and registrars, with several of the intervening days used to clear the cases needing operating time, ward rounds, more definitive later surgery and outpatient follow up and fracture clinics. It was a busy and stimulating environment. It also defined a way of giving 24 hour cover for emergencies, with a dedicated team and continuity in the management of injured hospitalised cases, from the entrance through to outpatient follow up with the same team. As a result, doctors knew their patients "in the round" in a way that can only be imagined in the modern health service.

One of the traditions of team three was the midnight suppers held on nights on call when the registrar collected a takeaway meal and the consultant supplied brown pharmacological two-litre Winchester bottles of cider. It was extremely rare for a critical patient to arrive after midnight, so the meal allowed the team to discuss the "take" of that day and learn lessons in a convivial environment.

Apart from the nurses and doctors, the staff of the hospital included a wide range of professions and specialties some of whom we have already met. Each group and every individual played a role in the holistic treatment offered to Birmingham's trauma victims. These multidisciplinary teams were truly pioneering in the 1940s and in most cases were not to be established for almost 50 years.

Sounding like a character from the *Canterbury Tales* and originally chaplains or church officers who were in charge of distributing money to the deserving poor, almoners (alms givers) were employed from 1945 and would nowadays be known as social workers. Uniquely, every BAH patient had access to an almoner.

Their aim was to ensure that patients made the best use of their abilities after discharge by facilitating access to community resources. In line with Gissane's principles, the ultimate goal was the best health that could be achieved and the maximum measure of independence. The department consisted of three almoners and two clerks. In addition, there were nearly always two almoner students training at the BAH who spent their time observing and undertaking medical-social casework. The almoners worked closely with the rehabilitation teams and an almoner was attached to each of the clinical teams – an early example of the sort of multidisciplinary working that would transform modern trauma care. The Burns Unit had its own dedicated almoner.

Rehabilitation was, and is, a key part of the management of anyone who has suffered significant trauma. An almoner met every patient as they attended the rehabilitation department for the first time to plan their recovery. They ensured that patients had the means to attend whatever follow up was deemed necessary, a not infrequent issue for those unable to work in the early post-war years. A man on workman's compensation shortly after the War might receive £2 10 0d a week; bus fares to the hospital of 9d per day, six days a week thus amounted to 4 shillings and sixpence (4/6) and represented a significant part of the family's available funds. Unusually, the hospital almoners also received referrals from the industries in which people worked, by ambulance personnel and by other staff within the hospital; they were also routinely informed of every hospital admission and discharge. The almoner worked to ensure a close and strong link between industry and the patient, liaising with the employer's personnel department to manage the problems of the returning worker.

Careful records of each patient's social needs were kept alongside their medical notes and the social and medical aspects of care were integral to each other. At the same time, detailed punch cards were used to store patient information including gender, accident type, source of referral, occupation and engagement with voluntary and state bodies. This data could then be used for research purposes and to aid in the development of services. The hospital almoners were also responsible for the supply of surgical appliances which, by the mid-1940s were available free of charge. Almoners also assisted in the finding of convalescence homes most suited to each patient; chest cases responded particularly well when sent to resorts on the warmer drier south coast.

The surgeons continued to push the boundaries of trauma treatment, although these years were not all plain-sailing. In 1947 two comments appear in the Medical Society records: that infection rates might reduce if a changing room was provided "*so that surgeons do not walk into theatre in ordinary clothes and outdoor shoes*" and that "*a reliable supply of cold water permitting scrubbing up without scalding of the hands in the process would do much to maintain the even temper of surgeons.*" In addition, the buildings were decrepit, often poorly suited to their function and the backlog of necessary repairs was long.

However, recognition of the BAH as a centre of excellence was not long in coming. The Hunterian Professorship and lecture of the Royal College of Surgeons are named after the pioneering surgeon-scientist John Hunter, and have been awarded annually by the Royal College of Surgeons of England since 1810 in recognition of a significant contribution to surgical or dental science. Previous winners have included many of the pioneers of British surgery. In the early 1950s the Hunterian Professorship was awarded to Accident Hospital clinicians for three years in succession, one of the winners being the ill-fated Peter Essex-Lopresti.

In 1947, Dr Simon Sevitt set up a pathology department that included the specialties of bacteriology (the study of infections), haematology (study of the blood and its components), biochemistry, histology (tissues under the microscope), and anatomy (post-mortem examinations). Simon Sevitt had won a scholarship to Trinity College, Dublin and had gained a host of academic prizes as an undergraduate. During the Second World War he served in East Africa as a military pathologist and at the hospital for head injuries in Oxford. Sevitt thrived at the BAH, establishing a multi-disciplinary clinical and research pathology department which undertook the whole range of pathology as it then existed: bacteriology, haematology, biochemistry, histology and morbid anatomy (gross anatomy of the human body). Nationally and internationally recognised in trauma research, his greatest contributions to patient care were in clarifying the importance of atherosclerosis, venous thrombosis (clots in the veins) and pulmonary embolism (blood clots in the lungs), and identifying the importance of prevention of blood clots following trauma. These breakthroughs were based on Sevitt's recognition of the high level of deaths from venous thrombosis and pulmonary embolism following surgery for a fractured femur. Sevitt's research interests covered a huge range of areas which would not be possible in the modern era of super-specialisation.

Sevitt also investigated fat embolism which occurs when fat from the marrow of broken bones enters the bloodstream causing blockages in blood vessels. He would later (1959) publish a paper on thromboembolism after fracture of the hip in the elderly which reported that fatal pulmonary embolism could occur as much as 30 days or more after surgery for hip fracture. This controversial paper resulted in a great deal of research interest and would eventually revolutionise the prevention, diagnosis and treatment of the condition. During his career at the BAH, as if this was not enough, Sevitt also produced important work on renal failure, burns and fracture healing. Contemporary medical students especially, but clinicians more generally, rarely attend post-mortem examinations of deceased patients. This is at least in part due to the fact that fewer such examinations are being carried out. This in turn is probably due to an unwillingness to ask grieving relatives for consent. A central element of traditional medical education and practice was regular attendance at such examinations and Sevitt believed implicitly that the correlation between clinical and pathological findings was an essential part of medical practice, especially when the precise cause of death was unclear.

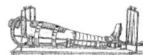

The later 1940s and 50s were, in many ways, the hospital's golden age. A tight-knit team was able to drive forward the care of the injured across a wide range of areas and disciplines and to develop an integrated pattern of medical and social care that would, it could be argued, not be equalled until the turn of the twenty-first century. In 1946 the unit investigating wound infection expanded its remit to include industrial skin diseases and was renamed the MRC Industrial Research Unit. New laboratories and a medical library were opened early in 1947 and remarkably ten beds were made available solely for research purposes.

The year after the War ended, the BAH saw a total of 4,757 new patients with a total of 94,682 attendances for follow up, further surgery, assessment and rehabilitation. The rehabilitation workshop, started at the Austin Motor Company in 1943, had returned over 800 employees to full time employment by the end of

4. State of the Art

1946. The following year physiotherapy, occupational therapy and remedial gymnastics were more closely co-ordinated to offer an integrated system and the Ministry of Health invited the department to assess a new electrotherapy unit for the treatment of peripheral nerve lesions. Physiotherapy and occupational therapy students from local hospitals were accepted for clinical training as well as physical education students from Bedford Physical Training College who attended for short periods to learn remedial exercises. In 1947, the hospital had 170 beds and an emergency department designed for 25,000 attendances a year, but which saw 34,000 (some things don't change). Extension plans were drawn up, but scrapped as a result of post-war building restrictions. The board commented in its report that they hoped *"that the springs of private charity may not dry up before the tides of public benevolence begin to flow"*, a reference to the new NHS, then called the Government Health Scheme, which was then in the offing. The total salary bill for the hospital at this time was £31,836 and for medical staff £17,193. This figure reflected the fact that in pre-NHS days consultants were expected to earn most of their income from private practice. Junior doctors were very poorly paid, a situation not properly addressed for almost 50 years.

The idea of a separate accident hospital was innovative and unique within the fledging National Health Service when it was established in 1948. Although it was already gathering plaudits for its exceptional trauma care, the isolation of the BAH from other acute specialties led to problems. For example, neurosurgery was not available at the BAH – it existed on its own in Smethwick – and although early brain-saving surgery could be carried out by the BAH surgeons, anything else either required the neurosurgeon to come to the BAH or a complex and potentially risky transfer of a critically injured patient. Similarly, if the patient had a coincidental medical problem, the expertise of a physician from one of Birmingham's other hospitals had to be sought, although this did not entail the same risk. Gissane planned to associate the hospital more closely with other specialist units but these plans had to be abandoned because of a lack of funds.

The National Health Service inherited a large number of casualty departments, many of them small, most of them in accommodation which was not fit for purpose and in poor condition. The standard of emergency care was generally poor and support from consultants, who were in nominal charge, was minimal: they were scathingly referred to as "absentee landlords" by one of the founders of modern emergency medicine. What began as casualty departments (staffed by casualty officers) would become accident and emergency departments (A&E) and finally emergency departments (ED). Departure from the current orthodoxy in correct use of terminology by older clinicians is likely to result in a pitying look from younger colleagues.

Because most of the departments were not planned or staffed adequately, the situation became more serious as they became busier and it was increasingly recognised that the level of care in the average casualty department was below an acceptable standard. The casualty department at the Accident Hospital, of course, served only the victims of trauma and, as a result, consultant cover could be provided by trauma surgeons who were either general surgeons or orthopaedic surgeons but were capable of operating on all forms of trauma whether to the bones, abdomen or chest. An aside about the nature of surgical practice is appropriate here and reflects issues which are as current in the third decade of the twenty-first century as they were in the early post-war years. The BAH's breed of trauma surgeons confident to operate on all forms of bodily trauma survived until the hospital's closure, but is now as extinct as Hugh Owen Thomas' forebear bone setters. In modern surgical practice, the role of the orthopaedic surgeon is apparent, cardiac or thoracic surgeons operate within the chest and general surgeons, by and large, within the abdomen. Historically, generally surgeons operated much more widely and were as at home surgically within the chest as elsewhere. As late as the 1980s, a general surgeon might ask for a chest case from his waiting list, as he hadn't done one for a while!

The term "general surgeon" survives, referring to the generality of abdominal surgeons, but most surgeons operating within the abdomen now have their own area of speciality whether it be the liver, kidneys or bowel. The true general surgeon, as Gissane would recognise the term, no longer exists. In the NHS this may be of little concern, because, as we shall see, major trauma centres were eventually established exactly to ensure that *all* the necessary specialists are available on-site. When it became necessary to ensure that surgeons deployed in small numbers to Iraq and Afghanistan had the capability to operate across body systems and regions, the issue of training modern surgeons to be capable and confident in dealing with a broad range of injuries outside their normal scope of practice became a major challenge which required innovative and ground-breaking solutions. This problem will remain current as long as there are no active conflicts allowing military surgeons to train in a combat zone and as long as there is no dedicated training programme for such surgeons.

In the 1940s, meanwhile, the Accident Hospital and its team of trauma surgeons was continuing to develop and refine the treatment of the critically injured. Let us consider the progress of a patient injured in an industrial accident in the early post-war years. Arriving at the hospital, the patient would enter the casualty department (debates about terminology were a thing of the future). The department was a long artificially lit room with curtained cubicles down one side (patient privacy was limited). There were integrated X-ray facilities and an operating theatre, as well as a room for dressings and a soundproof room. As the service continued to develop,

4. State of the Art

major trauma cases were taken straight to the Major Injuries Unit (MIU) via a separate entrance. The management of every serious casualty was led by a consultant, 24 hours a day, a model of care still not available in every one of our modern trauma centres, but one which has been proven to improve survival rates in the critically injured.

The Major Injuries Unit opened in 1959 and was the first resuscitation and intensive care unit in the UK to admit patients directly from the ambulance. The delightfully named Mr Badger, consultant trauma surgeon, was the driving force in the establishment of the unit. There was a dedicated telephone line into the unit from ambulance control. The unit accepted patients of all ages from infant to elderly, although it mainly dealt with adults and only rarely treated children. Then as now, serious trauma in the very young is fortunately rare. When it does occur, management in centres experienced in providing care to the smallest trauma patients is absolutely vital. Severely injured patients were met by a consultant trauma surgeon, a consultant anaesthetist and the medical and nursing teams. A radiographer was included in the initial alert and porters were on standby to move patients and to fetch blood and equipment. Consultants were present for almost all admissions and were on call with

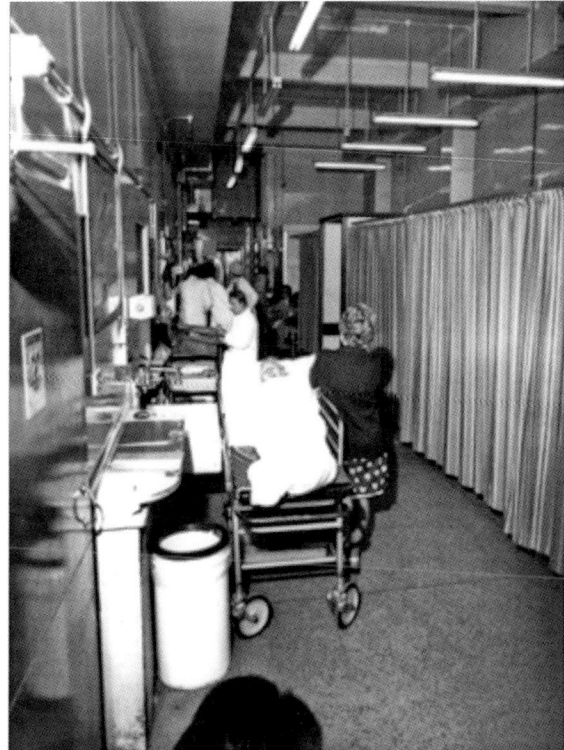

Casualty. This is an early photograph, but the department looked little different at the time of the hospital's closure.

their team 24 hours a day. The admitting medical team maintained responsibility for the care of the patient from arrival until discharge from outpatients and uniquely the nursing team, who were involved in resuscitating a patient, continued to look after them. The MIU also acted as the intensive care unit for the whole hospital and patients from the Burns Unit or the general trauma wards were transferred if their condition warranted high dependency or intensive care. Astonishingly by today's standards, there was usually an empty ward in the hospital which could be opened at short notice for the reception of multiple casualties (as well as providing a bed for exhausted medical students!). In times when the presence of the father was frowned upon during childbirth, and active family involvement in medical care was unusual, it is remarkable that patients' families were encouraged to be involved in all the stages of their relatives' resuscitation, treatment and rehabilitation from the earliest days of the Accident Hospital.

Throughout its life, the MIU would pioneer new medical interventions including arterio-venous haemofiltration as a means of treating kidney failure, extra-dural intracranial pressure monitoring and the treatment of multiple rib fractures with high thoracic epidural analgesia. The Institute of Accident Surgery (motto: *Tend and Mend*) was founded at the BAH and rapidly became recognised as the country's leading trauma research unit.

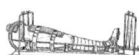

Edward Lowbury arrived in Birmingham in 1949 after Army service, mainly in East Africa and a period working for the Common Cold Research Unit alongside James Lovelock of Gaia fame. He was born in London, the son of Benjamin William Loewenberg (of Latvian-Jewish background) and his Brazilian wife Alice Sarah Hallé (who was of German-Jewish origin). The family name was anglicised to Lowbury at the start of the Great War. His father was a medical doctor and Edward's middle names were chosen in honour of the surgeon Joseph Lister, the pioneer in fighting operative infection: a prophetic choice as it turned out. Lowbury also has the unique distinction of being an acclaimed poet, publishing a number of collections, as well as an accomplished pianist and a founder member of the Birmingham Chamber Music Society. Whilst a student at Oxford he won both the Newdigate Prize for poetry and the Matthew Arnold Memorial essay prize.

Lowbury's poem entitled *August 10th, 1945 – The Day After*, written in Kenya, where he was serving as a pathologist in the Royal Army Medical Corps, concerned the dropping of the second atomic bomb on Nagasaki. In 1973 Lowbury delivered the 3rd Keats Memorial Lecture and in 1974 he was elected to the Royal Society of

Literature; he received an OBE in 1979. One of his poems, inspired by Sibelius' work *Tapiola* was, with the composer's enthusiastic approval, dedicated to him. We shall encounter Lowbury's poem on the closure of the Accident Hospital in due course.

His contributions to healthcare were also significant. A consultant for the World Health Organisation and the first clinician to carry out clinical trials in burns treatment, he developed a laboratory test for surgical and hygienic hand disinfection in the 1960s, and later demonstrated the effectiveness of alcohol solutions in surgical hand disinfection and the value of silver-based compounds as topical antibacterial dressings. These developments continue to inform basic hygiene measures in these post-COVID days. Lowbury was also a founder and first president of the Hospital Infection Society and, with John Babb, confirmed and developed Colebrook's work on air filtration as a means of reducing hospital infections by eliminating bacteria. He was also a pioneer in the study of antibiotic resistance.

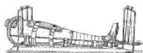

By the end of the 1950s and the beginning of the 60s, the Birmingham Accident Hospital was firmly recognised not only as a centre of excellence for the treatment of the victims of trauma, but also as a world-leading centre for research, especially in the treatment of burns and the management of hospital acquired infection. Its model of integrated multidisciplinary care was established and the distinction of its staff made them sources of advice both nationally and internationally. The BAH's management of the injured patient followed a series of simple principles, articulated by Gissane and his colleagues and based on experience, successes and failures and sound scientific principles. The treatment of shock was based on early accurate diagnosis of the injury or injuries which required urgent surgical treatment, with the aim of resuscitating the patient until they were fit for surgery. This surgery was to be carried out by a senior and experienced surgeon. Open fractures with skin loss, still often seen in motorcycle accident injuries to the legs, were closed using a number of grafting techniques after careful surgical cleansing in order to prevent wound infection, provide adequate skin cover and expedite return to the best achievable function. Leonard Colebrook had proved that the longer a wound remains open the more certain it is to become infected.

The shock associated with severe burns and scolds was treated with blood plasma and scrupulous attention to sterile dressings, which were used to reduce the risk of infection. Wounds were covered with grafts as soon as safely possible and attention was paid to the nutritional status of the patient, an aspect of care often still forgotten in trauma cases. Limbs were splinted in a position of function to promote rehabilitation and prevent contractures and deformity. These basic principles, which remarkably were not widely accepted until relatively recently, ensured that the Accident Hospital had the best outcomes for any similar group of patients in the country.

The aseptic room in which the patients had their burns dressed was unique at the time. A constant stream of filtered fresh air was directed into the room by an electric fan, while open culture-plates were exposed at different parts of the room so that, if any bacteria grew on them it would be possible to trace it to its source by bacteriological examination of every person who was known to be in the room at the time of dressing the wound. As a result, the most effective antibiotic could be identified.

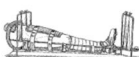

With much of the Midland's heavy industry still in operation, hand injuries were common and had potentially devastating consequences for wage-earners, especially in highly-skilled manual trades. Such injuries were treated early in their course, and always, of course, by experienced specialist surgeons. The best results were achieved by surgery in stages and obsessive attention to the risk of infection and its treatment were key components of the approach. Unsurprisingly, fractures of all kinds formed the largest group of patients treated by the hospital. These were managed with close attention to detail, careful manipulation, and in the early days at least, most often immobilisation in traction or in plaster of Paris. As with all significant injuries, effective and intense rehabilitation was essential.

Patients were admitted or attended with injuries of varying degrees of severity and were divided according to their clinical needs in the casualty department. Inevitably the hospital increasingly began to see patients transferred from other hospitals. Gissane, the founder of the concept of a specialist trauma hospital, was able to conclude that it *"has convinced me of its rightness."* He described the "surgery of function", meaning treatment intended to maximise the functional outcomes for the patient. Gissane was so certain of his vision that he felt that the skills and experience it offered should be shared with those of other, smaller, less specialist hospitals. As part of this, and in accordance with his mantra of multidisciplinary engagement, he promoted friendly and close relationships with elective orthopaedics, plastics, maxillofacial surgery and a multitude of professional specialists, including members of all the key professions essential to optimal patient care. Although it sounds obvious now, at the time it was in marked contrast to the inter-specialist rivalries so memorably captured by the irascible surgeon Sir Lancelot Spratt and the effete physician personified by Kenneth Williams. In this great tradition of consultant eccentricity one of the BAH's surgeons, James (Jim) Edward Morgan Smith, had the endearing habit of referring to patients who were disobedient or troublesome as "bounders". Incidentally, a condition of his employment was that his home had to be within walking distance of the hospital.

Reference has already been made to the treatment of children, especially those with burns. The children's ward was Ward 1, a traditional nightingale ward, with, by night, the nurses sitting at one end in the light of a desk light which allowed all the patients to be observed and a suitably child-friendly atmosphere to be promoted. There was a small area for play and teaching and a number of single rooms for the patients that needed them.

Careful written guidance was offered to the parents of small patients, it began: "*We are sorry that your child has had an accident and hope he* [sic] *will soon be well again. We shall give him every attention and the best possible treatment, but you, too, will want to play your part in helping him to get better, and there is much you can do.*"

There was a definite flavour of the early post-war years about the subsequent advice which included: "*Do try to be calm when you are with him and go quickly at the end of visiting time. At first he may cry when you leave, but it is better that he should do this, and learn that you will come again, than feel he is deserted because you do not come.*"

Not to mention: "*ALWAYS TELL YOUR CHILD THE TRUTH* [their original capitals] *... and do not promise to come again later if you know you cannot do this ... You should know how your child is progressing. Enquire about your child's progress at least once a week* [!] *from the ward sister or one of the doctors. The doctors wear a red label on their white coats denoting consultant surgeon, registrar or house surgeon. Tell sister about any food fads, his special word for toilet and if he likes a special toy for going to sleep.*"

Advice was also offered regarding life after discharge: "*Your child may be cross, irritable and demanding, or he may cling constantly to you and not let you out of sight ... Frequent extra love and attention, (though he is trying your patience to the limit) is enough to help him settle down again.*" Unfortunately, advice was not offered regarding how to distinguish this behaviour from that of the average toddler.

The hospital was legally required to provide education for children. Within a few days of admission and once they were well enough to take part, they would be visited daily by one of the hospital teachers. The teaching was tailored to the individual child, taking into account their age and ability, and special arrangements were made to help those such as burns victims who had little or no use of their hands; liaison with each child's school was close. Like adult patients, children were encouraged to take part in crafts.

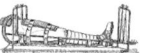

As it had from its earliest days, as the post-war decades passed, research into improving patient care remained at the heart of the Accident Hospital's mission; over 1,000 research papers would eventually be published by the small staff of the Accident Hospital. Trauma related infection remained a key area of interest as it had been since high levels of infection had been observed in the survivors of Dunkirk. It had been established that apart from the time immediately after injury, the most common time for a wound to become infected after surgery was when it was being dressed. Research at the Wound Infection Unit would establish the now universal "no touch" technique for wound dressing. The research opportunities offered by the availability of large numbers of trauma patients at a single specialist hospital were widely recognised.

The Road Injuries Research Group was a pioneering unit established by Dr John Bull and Professor William Gissane at the suggestion of Dr Donald Stewart, the chief medical officer at the Austin Motor Company and a member of the governing body of the AA, which provided the initial funding. Much of the early data was collected by Miss Barbara Roberts who collated all the fatal accidents in and around Birmingham in 1960. This amounted to 149 people who died on the city's streets and another 34 fatalities brought into Birmingham from the surrounding areas. It should be remembered that at this time there were no seatbelts and safety features in cars and other vehicles were largely non-existent. The group published its first report in 1961 with a number of hard-hitting recommendations for vehicle safety. Their recommendations included the importance of the car's exterior being smooth, without projections where possible, in order to lessen the severity of injuries caused by direct impact between the vehicle and pedestrians or cyclists. The report also recommended that bumpers should be wide and deep, and covered with energy absorbing material to lessen the severity of direct impacts, and that number plates should be flush fitting. In addition, the report recommended that vehicle doors should be hollow and filled with energy absorbing plastic for the protection of car occupants against side-on impacts, most commonly at road junctions. The Road Injuries Research Group would also emphasise the importance of protective measures such as helmets and seatbelts. The culture of data gathering and analysis would in the future provide the basis for road safety legislation and the hospital would work closely with the Government Road Research Organisation.

The third in the trinity of major research units at the Accident Hospital was the Industrial Medicine Unit which was formed by Professor John Squire in 1946; on Leonard Colebrook's retirement in 1948 it merged with the Burns Unit to form the

4. State of the Art

Industrial Medicine and Burns Research Unit which John Squire led until he moved to Birmingham University in 1952, at which time Dr John Bull became director and the unit was renamed The Industrial Injuries and Burns Unit, thus proving that serial renaming is not a new health service phenomenon. John Bull's medical training had been interrupted by war service in the Royal Army Medical Corps. In 1947 he joined the staff of the Medical Research Council (MRC) Industrial Injuries and Burns Unit at Birmingham Accident Hospital. His research interests included road and vehicle safety (he was a founder of the hospital's Road Injury Research Group) and burns. In researching burn injury, he often used himself as an experimental subject.

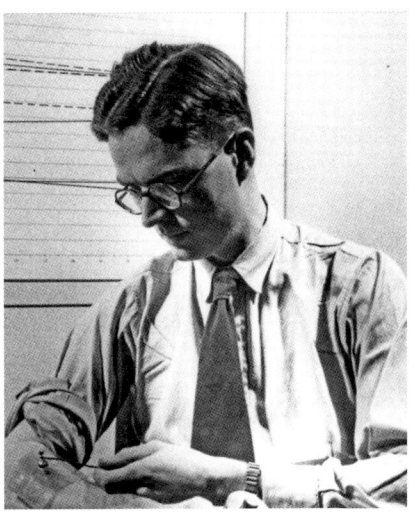

Dr John Bull carrying out investigations into burn thickness on himself.

As well as serving as chairman of the committee on road safety of the Medical Commission on Accident Prevention and chair of a laboratory trials group of the Ministry of Health, John Bull was an early advocate of cycling helmets, the single most important intervention in reducing cycling related deaths.

Following Colebrook's lead, the unit remained at the forefront of research into infection and in particular its relation to trauma. At the same time research also led to developments in blood transfusion for burns patients and new techniques for skin grafting, a process essential to the recovery of those with severe burns. The close relationship between industry and the Accident Hospital continued through the 1950s and 60s, even as clouds gathered over the Midland's huge manufacturing concerns and especially over the motor industry. An early research area was the treatment of the apparently minor hand injuries and infections which could still prevent a successful return to work. Once the unit had joined with the burns research unit, a wide range of issues was addressed, including the development of the first mortality tables for burns patients, which related the size of the burns a patient had suffered to the likelihood of their survival. At the same time, researchers were developing ways of determining the volumes of blood needed by patients with burns and other injuries, working with a newly established blood bank largely staffed by volunteers. Reflecting later developments in its management, which we will consider in due course, shock was perceptively referred to as "the illness of trauma". Post-mortem examination was also employed as a way of determining not only the immediate cause of death, but also of identifying other contributing issues such as blood clots. The effects of blood loss on the body were described in terms of naked eye assessment but also under the microscope. As a result, the effects of trauma on body systems were clarified and described. Attendance at post-mortem examinations was encouraged, from medical students to consultants as these occasions were considered a great teaching opportunity; one now almost entirely absent from medical education.

All these streams of research directly or indirectly influenced patient care at the hospital which, in the early days of the NHS, was under the direct control of its senior staff. As the health service grew and became more complex, this clinical oversight of the running of the hospital would inevitably decrease. Although it was always easier in a speciality hospital, the ability of clinicians to shape and direct the practical philosophy of the hospital in which they work is largely a thing of the past, lost to government directives, central guidance, legislation, targets and dictat.

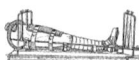

By the late 1950s clinical life at the BAH followed a familiar pattern. Each team alternated days on call, in outpatients and in the operating theatre. The previous day's X-rays were reviewed each morning by a consultant. The three surgical teams and all other medical staff attended the monthly meetings at which complex cases were reviewed and experts from outside the hospital came to speak. Teaching remained a key activity and by the 1950s the hospital was running not only the industrial nursing course established during the War, but also a course for industrial medical officers and a national course on the care of the injured which would run until 1990.

The Institute of Accident Surgery promoted education to the military, medical students, nursing students, physiotherapy and occupational therapy students. The result was a dynamic, engaging teaching environment. In due course, as well as trainee surgeons from the West Midlands, clinical training would be offered to military "medics" from the Special Air Service Regiment (SAS) and Parachute Regiment and refresher courses were offered for personnel deploying to the Falklands War in 1982.

The 1959 British Orthopaedic Association's *Memorandum on Accident Services* recommended that regional hospital boards, in association with the boards of teaching hospitals, set up at least one comprehensive accident service within their area. It was hoped that such units would integrate to form a nationwide accident service. However, the British Orthopaedic Association were in favour of having accident units that were part of a general hospital. It was recommended that these units be in the charge of orthopaedic surgeons as bones, joints and muscles accounted for three quarters of all injuries.

4. State of the Art

In practice it would be 50 years before anything like a coordinated accident service would be established, but in retrospect these recommendations can be seen as the first step on the way to establishing properly staffed Accident and Emergency Departments and then major trauma centres. The need for change was reinforced in 1960 by the Nuffield Provincial Report which showed that the casualty services in the studied areas were still badly housed in unplanned accommodation with inadequate staffing and minimal support from consultants for junior staff. Patients were generally dissatisfied with the experience of attending A&E and only the casualty sisters appeared to be appreciated! Further change was inevitable and in the early 60s the Platt Report would make the recommendations which would finally lead to something like a national emergency service and the establishment of accident and emergency medicine (now emergency medicine) as a speciality in its own right. Specialist trauma centres would remain a long way in the future.

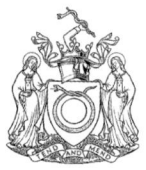

Second Interlude

Why do Trauma Patients Die?

WERE ONE TO be in the position to ask a surgeon at Waterloo or Balaclava, or on the battlefields of Normandy in 1944, what the commonest cause of death was following trauma, there is no doubt that the answer would be: bleeding. Trauma patients bleed to death. As was established beyond any doubt in Afghanistan, this remains true of battlefield trauma today and makes it all the more remarkable that tourniquets, long recognised as an effective means of controlling haemorrhage, and thus saving lives, not only had to be reintroduced into clinical practice during that conflict, but that their reintroduction was, at least in some quarters, controversial.

Most people, of course, do not die on the battlefield, although in some war-torn and violence ridden states, civilian trauma deaths follow a pattern aligned to that of conflict as violence becomes endemic amongst the civilian population. In 2021, worldwide 2,492 people were killed and 4,561 wounded by land mines. Sadly, terrorist incidents are now also a part of modern life, and as the tragic events in London in 2005 and Manchester in 2017 proved, injuries more typical of the battlefield do occur in civilian practice and victims do bleed to death. In civilian trauma, although the causes of death are more complex and death from bleeding is rare, the causes of most deaths are still entirely predictable from the nature of the injuries suffered. It goes without saying that an understanding of the nature of a patient's injuries and how they might cause a patient's demise is essential if the best possible treatment is to be offered. Much of the early work on understanding the effects of trauma on the human body was, as we have seen, carried out at the

Second Interlude

Birmingham Accident Hospital. It remains a fact, however, that research into the effects and management of trauma still does not attract a fraction of the funding allocated to conditions such as cancer or chronic neurological diseases. Such research breakthroughs, as there are, remain the result of the commitment and drive of individual researchers.

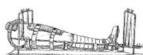

In 1976, an American trauma surgeon called James K. Styner, crashed his light aircraft in a field in Nebraska. His wife Charlene was killed instantly and three of his four children sustained critical injuries. His fourth child was luckier and only suffered a broken arm. Styner carried out the initial assessment of his children at the site of the crash. He then flagged down a car to transport him to the nearest hospital which was closed when he arrived. The hospital was eventually opened, but even then, the emergency treatment provided was unacceptably substandard. Having returned home Dr Styner declared: *"When I can provide better care in the field with limited resources than what my children and I received at the primary care facility, there is something wrong with the system and the system has to be changed"*.

As a result of his experiences, Styner would establish a course designed to train doctors to manage the victims of major trauma. It ran first in the USA and then spread across the world: it was called Advanced Trauma Life Support (ATLS) and its effects were transformational. Although it has been replaced by other courses (at least on this side of the Atlantic), its principles are at the heart of modern trauma care and can be used as our guide for a tour through the potential causes of death after trauma.

The precise details of the course have been adjusted in the light of experience and to fit local circumstances, but Styner's basic approach has saved countless lives: it is that traumatic injuries cause death in a largely predictable sequence and must, therefore, be managed in that sequence to maximise the chances of survival.

In establishing his course, Styner described the ABCDE sequence: Airway (A), Breathing (B), Circulation (C), Disability (D) and Exposure (E). Recent experience, especially of war injuries and injuries associated with terrorist attacks, has caused another C, this time a small c, to be added at the beginning to create cABCDE, but external haemorrhage severe enough to cause rapid death by exsanguination is sufficiently rare in civilian practice, outside of terrorist attacks, for this "small c" to be generally name-checked only, before moving on to more relevant areas.

By the time Dr Styner began his campaign to improve trauma care, the influence of Birmingham Accident Hospital had also spread to the USA. Having emigrated to the United States, a BAH alumnus, Professor Howard Champion, became one of the pioneers of a new generation of US trauma surgeons offering an entirely new standard of trauma care across the country based on Styner's ABCDE, but having at its heart the multidisciplinary team and senior clinical leadership developed and perfected by the BAH. Professor Champion arrived at the Shock Trauma Unit at the University of Maryland in Baltimore, one of the country's premier trauma centres, to find R. Adams Cowley, himself a distinguished trauma pioneer, *"screaming at a hoard of individuals surrounding trauma patients that had been admitted directly from the heliport or ambulance to an intensive care unit bed without any structural process to guide or secure their care"*. As a result, he introduced the team system and multidisciplinary training and reproduced a resuscitation area based on the one he had seen working so well in Birmingham. Within a few years he was able to reproduce this approach in Washington DC and eventually to see it spread to many leading trauma centres across America. Under Professor Champion's leadership, his Washington unit acquired a helipad and ambulance ramp with direct access to the resuscitation bays and operating rooms just as at the Birmingham Accident Hospital and a separate entrance from that used by the walking wounded at the emergency department. The introduction of these changes, based on the BAH model, in combination with Styner's innovations, would, as a network of trauma centres developed, eventually lead to significant improvement in trauma mortality across the USA. In time Professor Champion would work with American academic bodies to promulgate clinical standards from Birmingham which would eventually recross the Atlantic, with Styner's course, to influence British trauma care more widely and to break down the barriers between resuscitation, surgery and intensive care just as he had seen in Birmingham.

Setting aside the additional "c" for massive bleeding, Styner's approach begins with "A" for airway, evidence demonstrating that a blocked airway is the fastest cause of death following trauma, and consequently the issue that must be addressed first. (Incidentally, in surgical circles ABCD, is said to stand for Assess, Blame, Criticise and Deny). Patients who have suffered facial trauma may have blocked airways due to their tongue falling backwards, blood, damaged facial structures (bits of bone) or vomit (especially if they have been drinking). The first task of the rescuer therefore is to ensure a clear airway so that oxygen can pass into the lungs. This may involve suction of the airway and with positioning the patient so that fluids run out of the mouth and the tongue falls forwards, may be all that is required. In some cases, more advanced techniques are needed including anaesthesia and the passage of a tube into the trachea (windpipe), very occasionally it is necessary to insert a tube through a hole in the front of the neck, although most stories of such heroic "saves" using biros and other improvised equipment are apocryphal. Sadly, people still die from a blocked airway which may be easily treated.

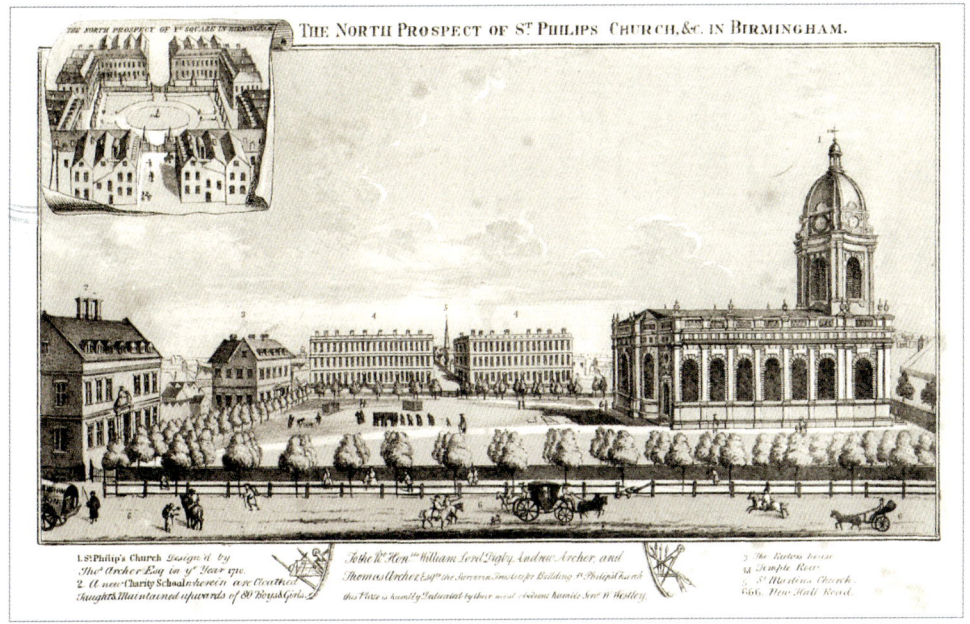

Eighteenth-century Birmingham with St Phillip's Church on the right and Temple Row in the background.

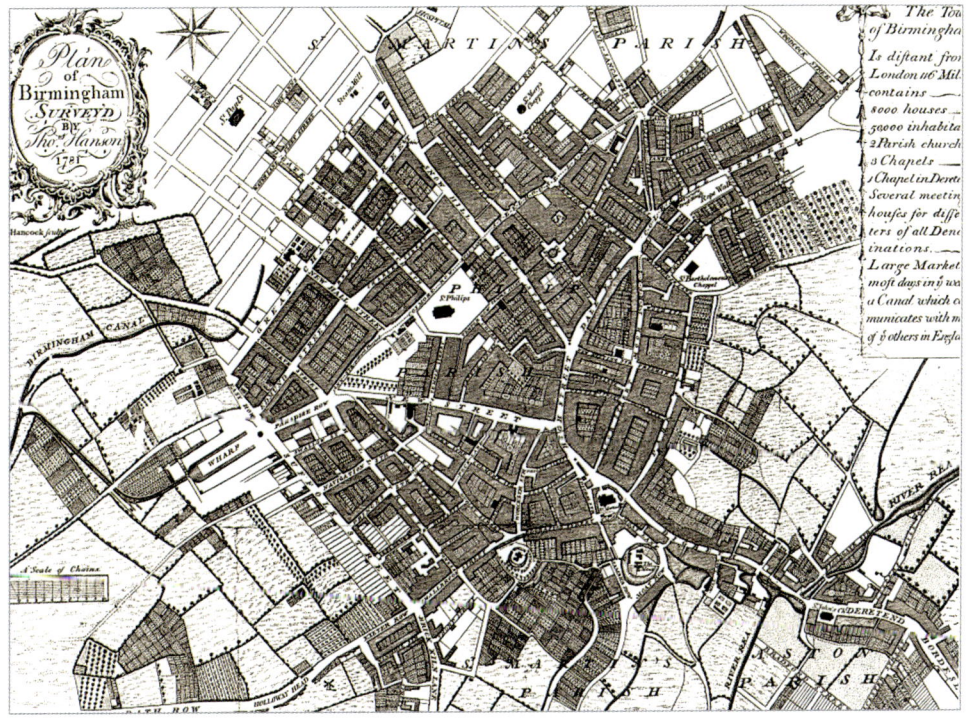

Birmingham 1781, Bath Row, site of the Queen's Hospital is at the bottom left.

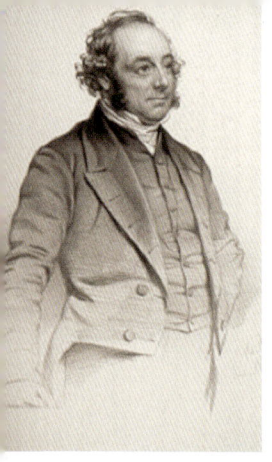 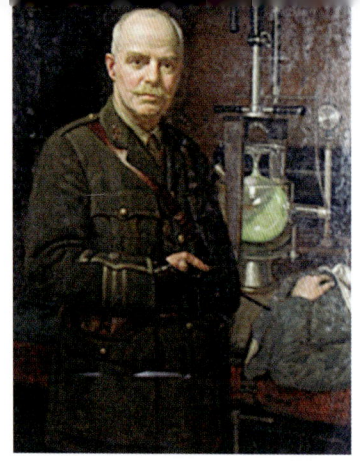 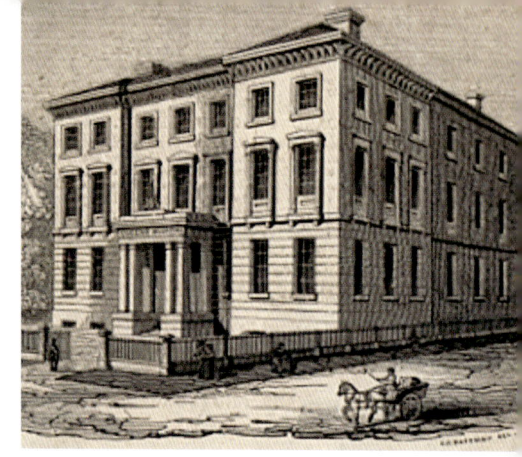

Above left: William Sands Cox FRCS FRS.

Above middle: Dr John Hall Edwards, pioneer of radiology and radiation safety. The portrait clearly shows the loss of Hall's left arm and the fingers of his right hand.

Above right: The Queen's Hospital.

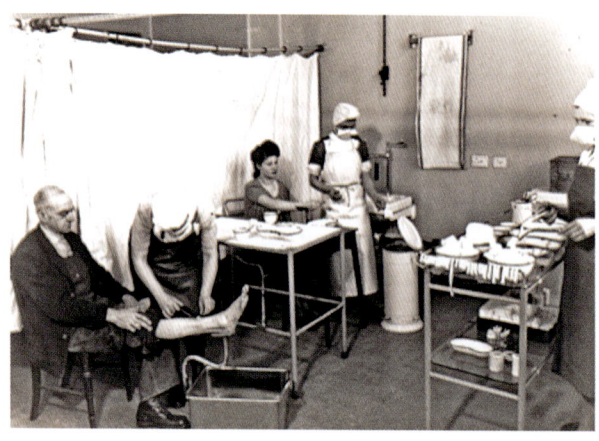

Left: The outpatients' department.

Below: A wedding on the ward.

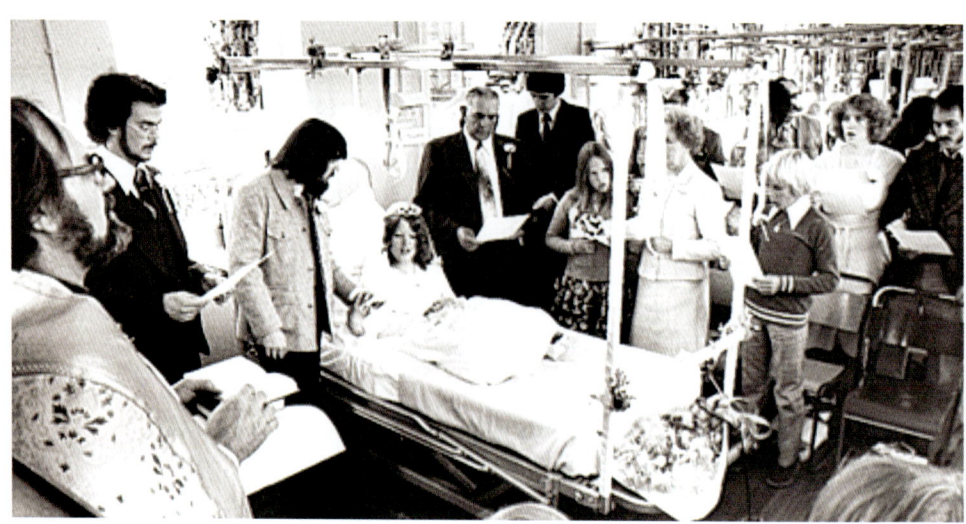

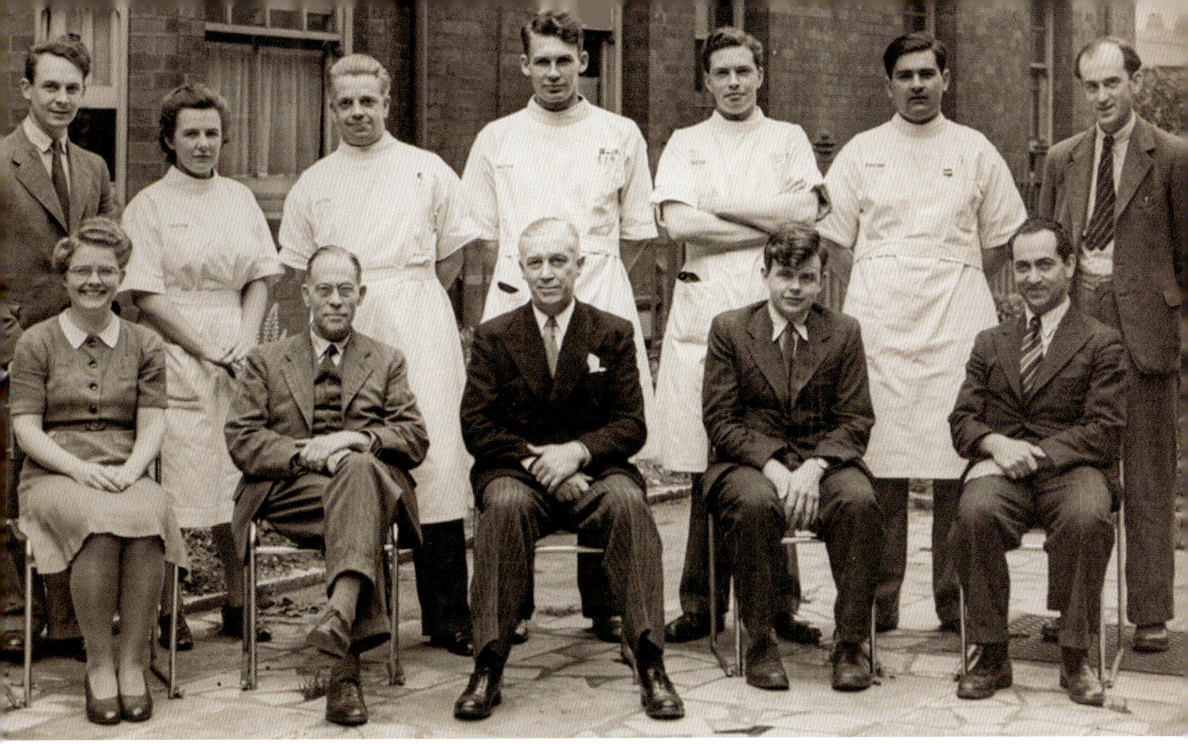

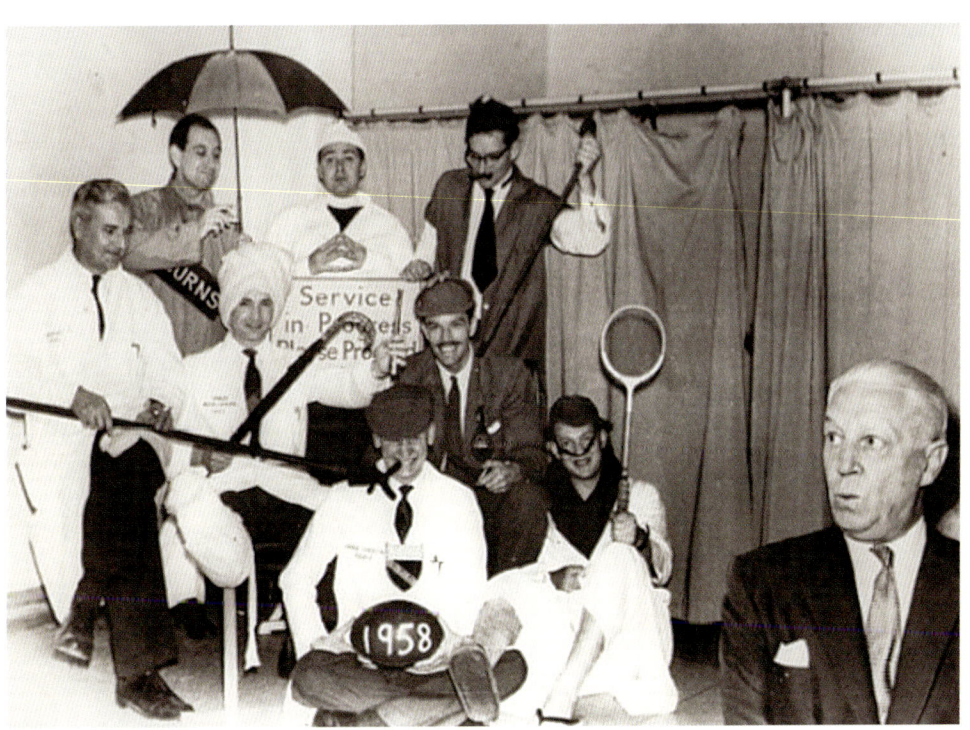

Accident Hospital Medical Staff 1945. "Colonel" Leonard Colebrook and William Gissane front row second and third from left.

Memories of a Christmas Show – a startled looking William Gissane bottom right.

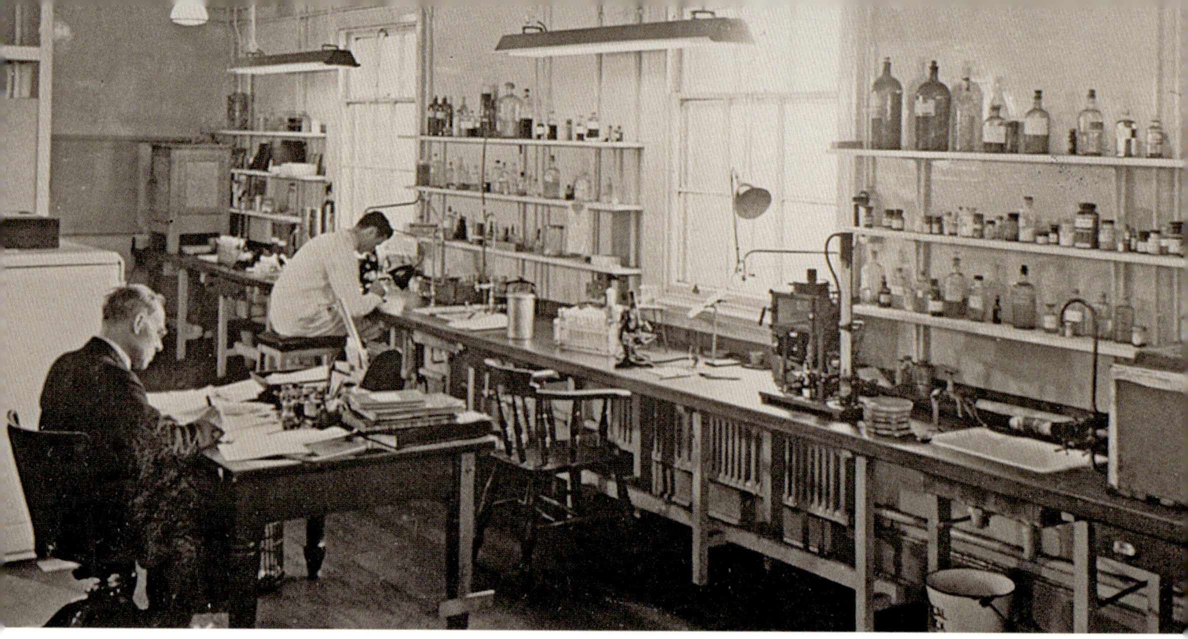

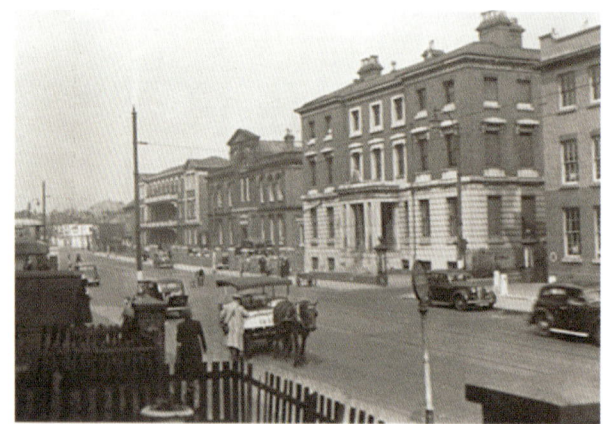

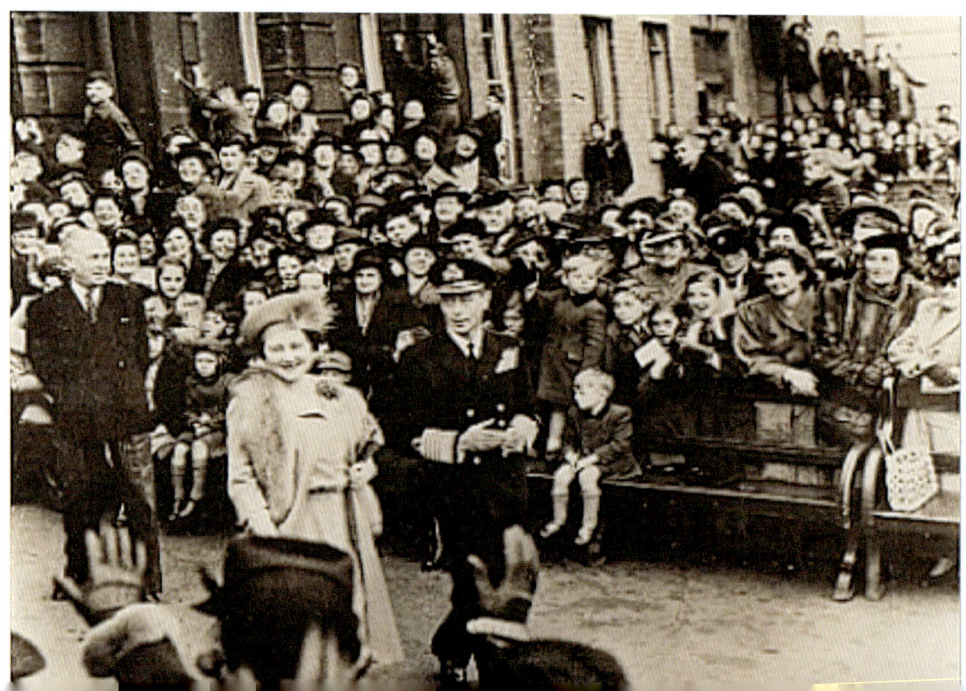

Above: The hospital laboratory.

Left: The Queen's Hospital, an early twentieth-century view.

Below: HM King George VI and Queen Elizabeth visit the Accident Hospital, 7th November 1945.

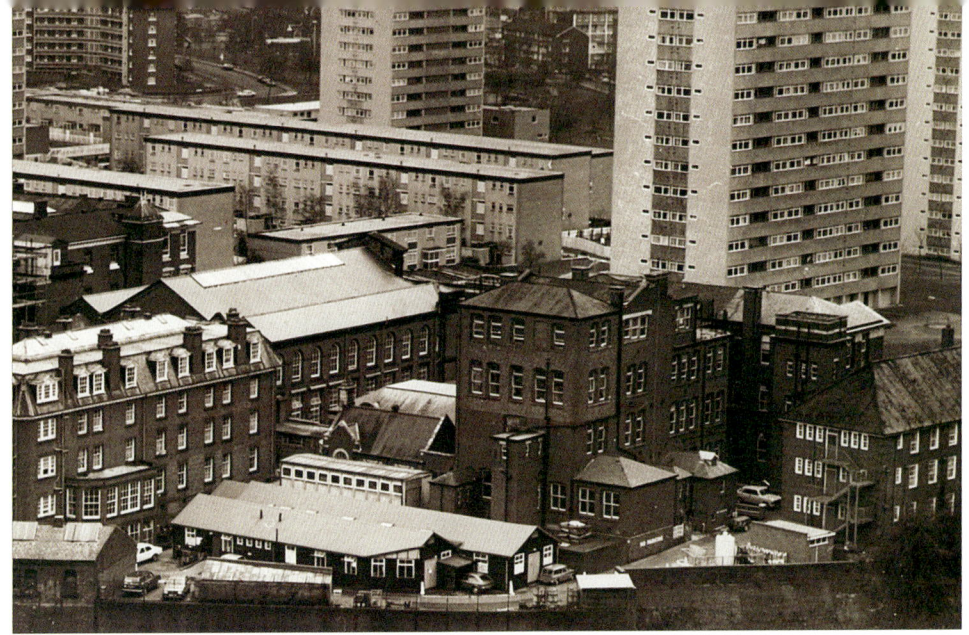

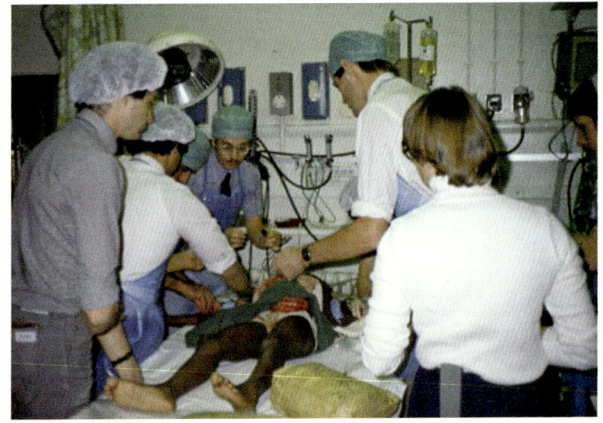

Above: The Acci from the air.
Right: A major trauma resuscitation.
Below: Dressing Clinic.

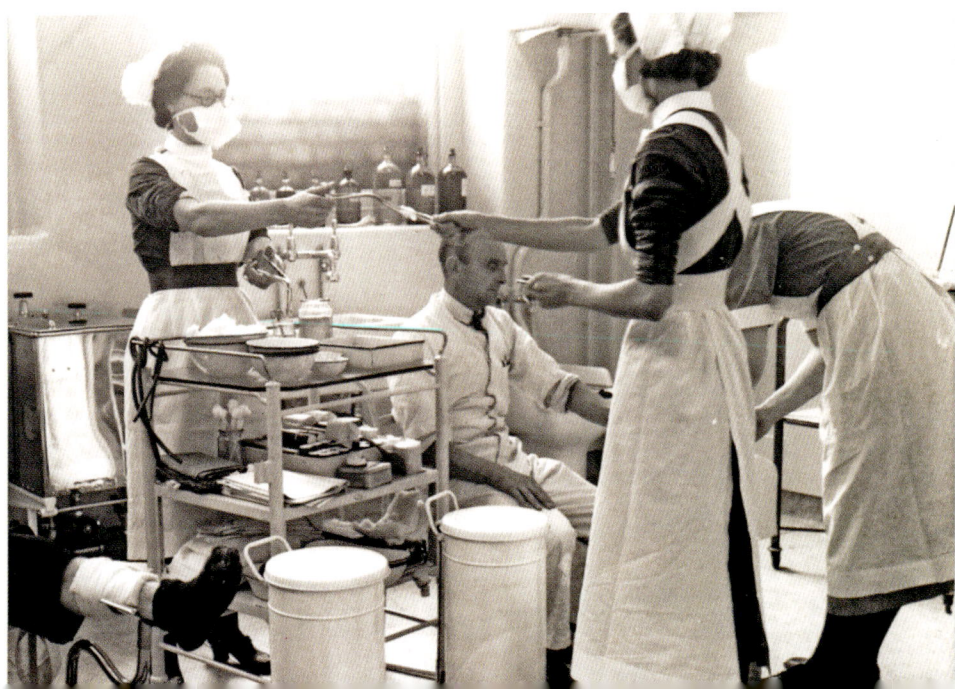

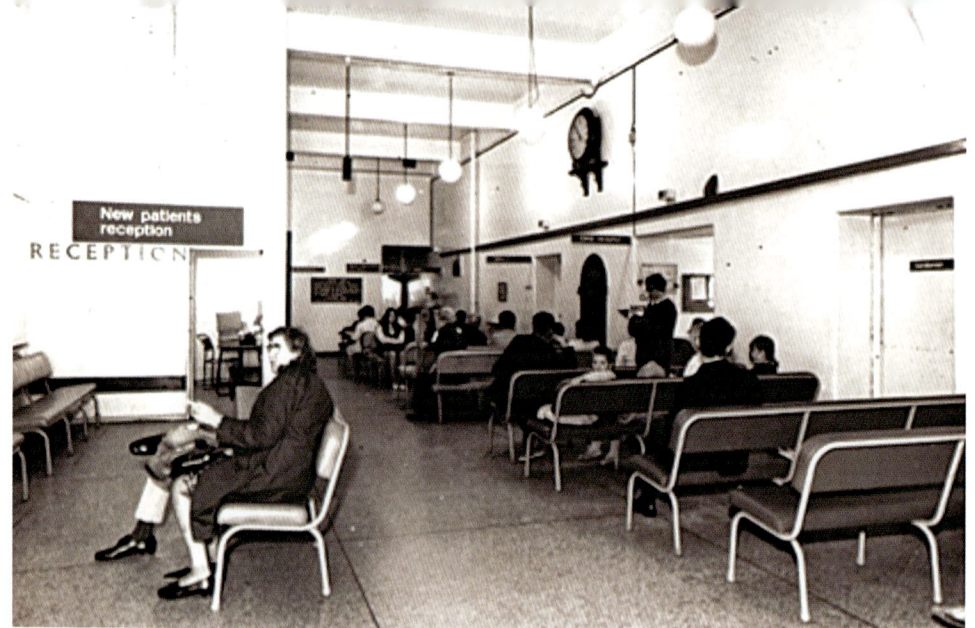

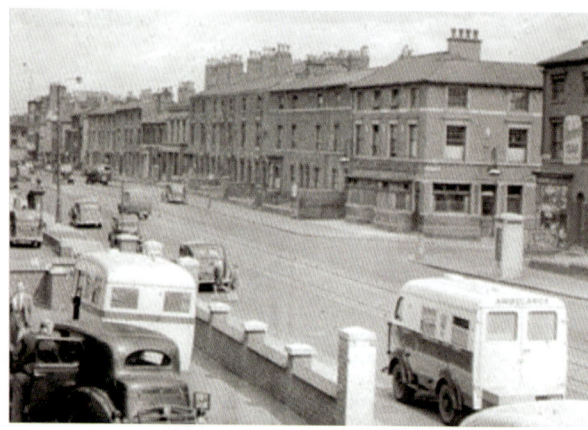

Above: The Acci waiting room.
Left: Bath Row from the BAH forecourt.
Below: The Children's Ward.

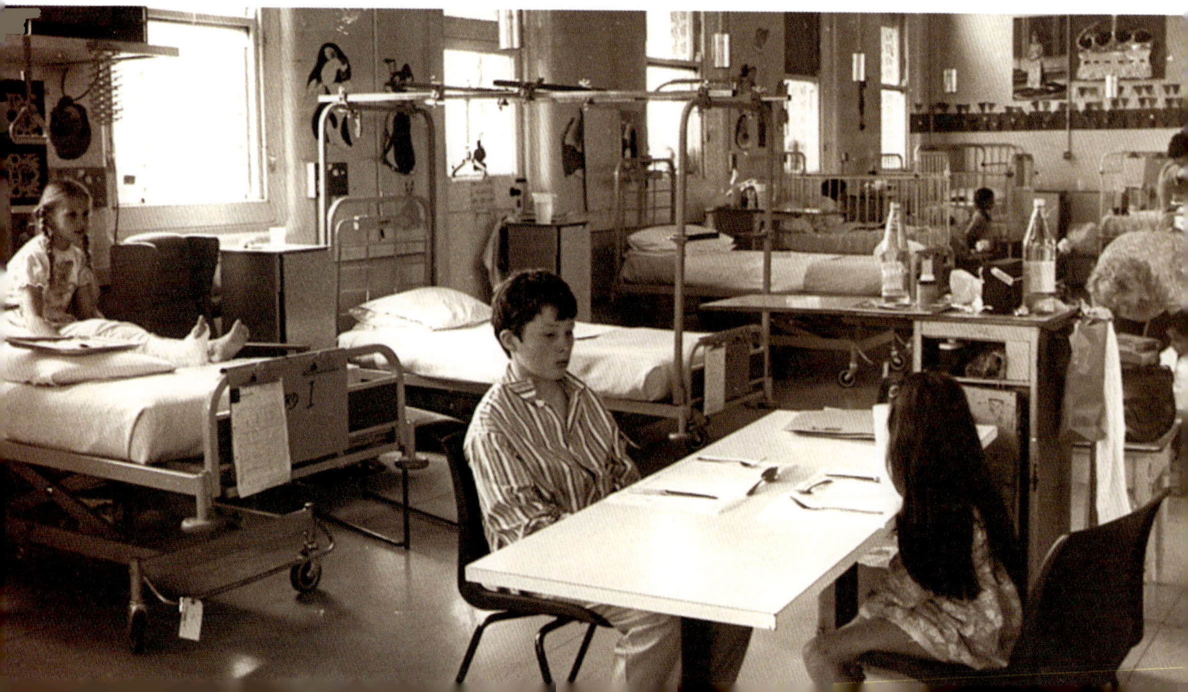

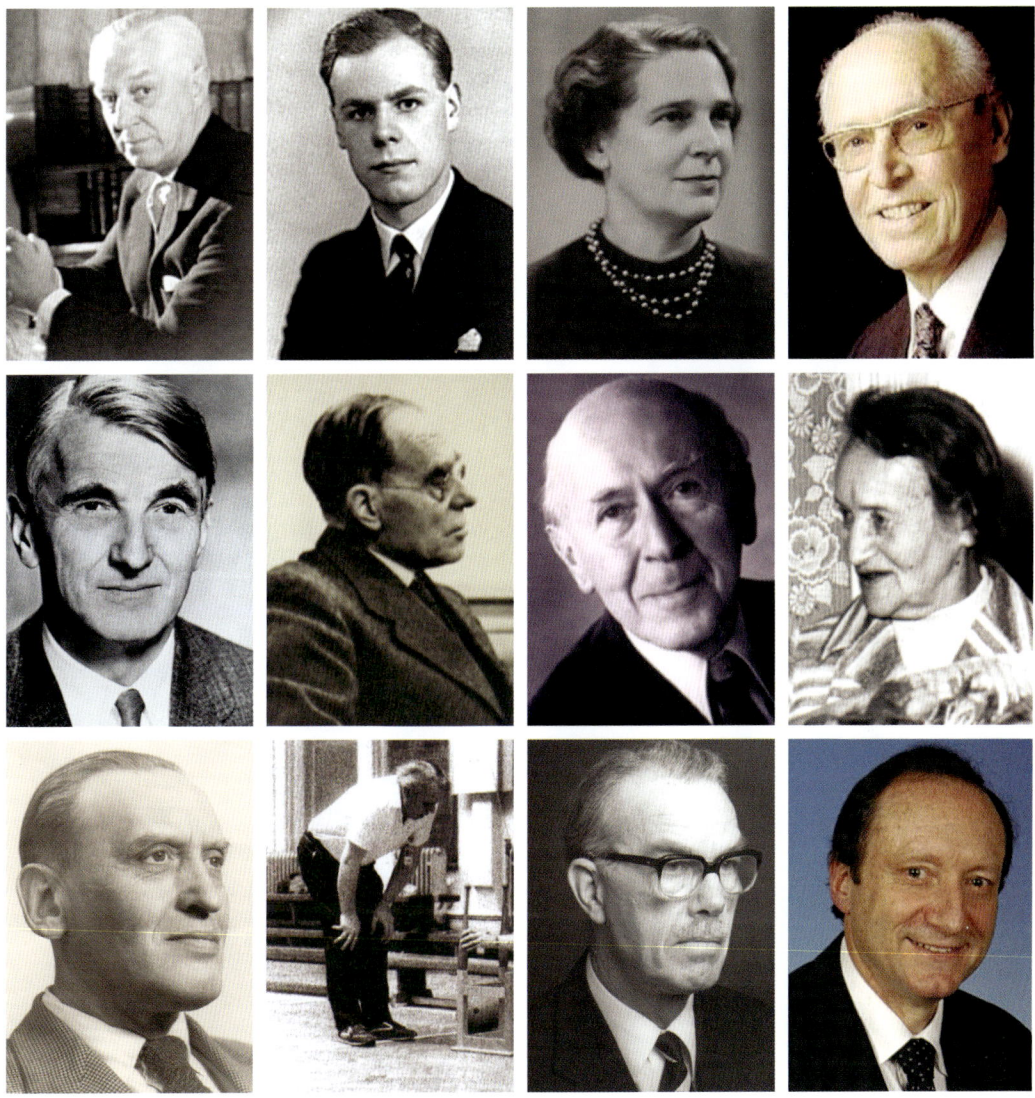

Top row: William Gissane CBE, Peter Essex-Lopresti, Ethel Florey, Douglas MacGilchrist Jackson.
Middle row: Sir Ashley Miles, Leonard Colebrook, Edward Lowbury OBE, Olga Muller.
Bottom row: Ruscoe Clark MBE, Jack Thackeray, Peter London MBE, Sir Keith Porter.

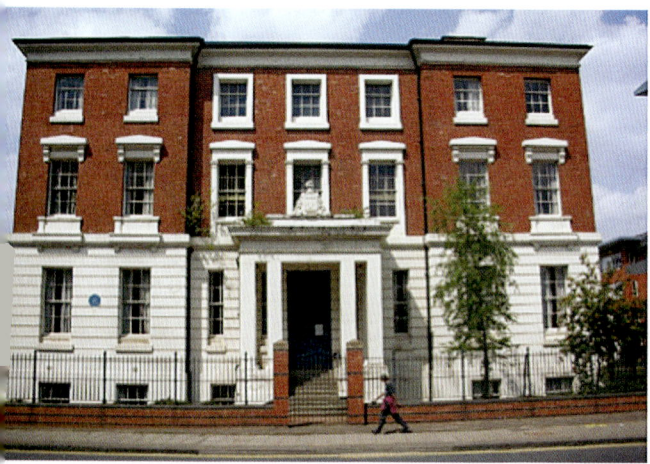
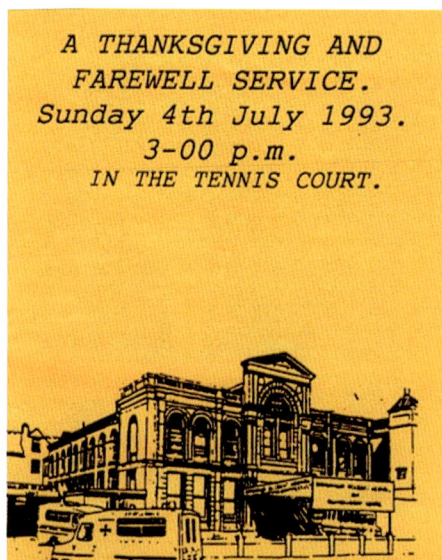
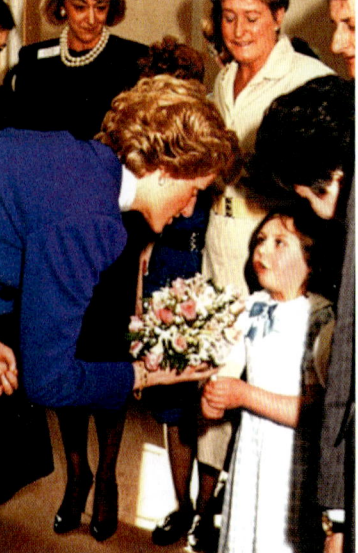

Above left: The Birmingham Accident Hospital in retirement.

Above right: Programme for the Birmingham Accident Hospital farewell service.

Left: The visit of HRH Diana, Princess of Wales.

Right: The air ambulance lands.

Below: The Queen Elizabeth Hospital, Birmingham.

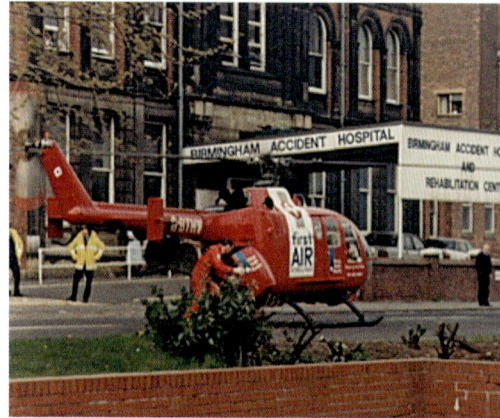
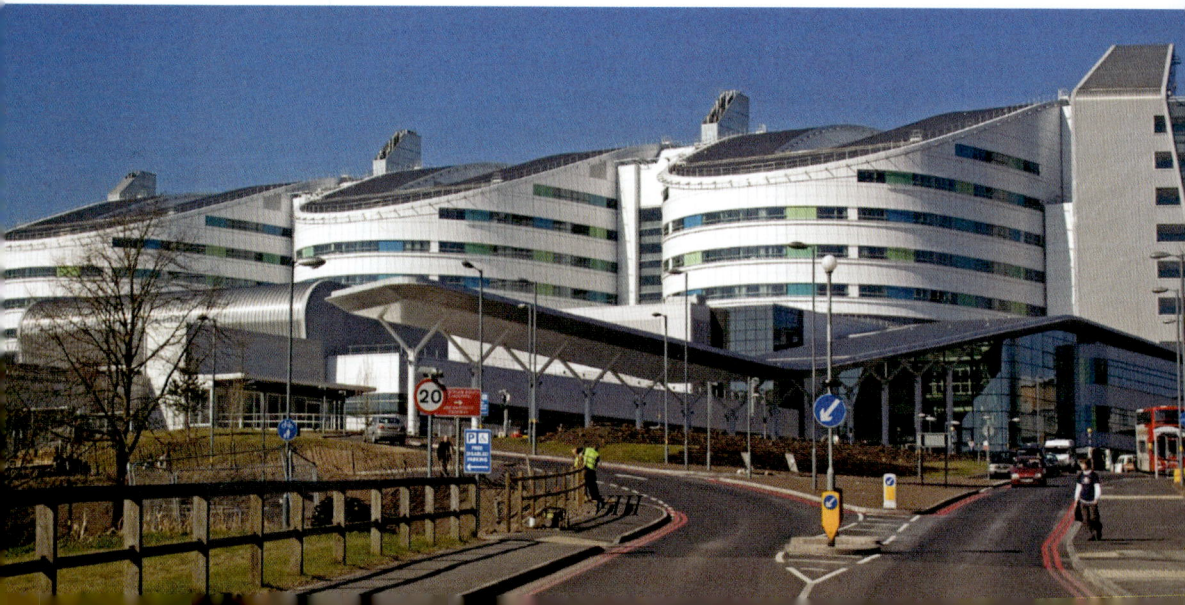

Second Interlude

The next step "B" – breathing – is the management of chest injuries with the aim of ensuring that oxygen delivered to the lungs via an open airway can be effectively absorbed into the bloodstream. Injuries identified here include collapsed lungs, bleeding inside the chest and holes in the chest wall allowing air to enter into the chest (but not the lung) from outside and, in turn, causing the lung to collapse. In most cases simple treatment is effective and lifesaving. A hole can be made in the wall of the chest and a tube inserted to allow the drainage of air and blood; lost blood can be replaced. Rarely, if the patient has suffered a cardiac arrest, it may be necessary to open the chest itself to control internal bleeding from a hole in the heart (for example from a stab-wound) or damage to one of arteries to the lungs. In very severe cases blood can be administered directly into the heart. In most cases blood is given via a needle into a vein and the technique of intraosseous infusion, where blood is given via a needle into the marrow of a major bone, brought into widespread clinical practice after military use in Afghanistan, offers an alternative in small children or where a vein cannot be used.

The "C" stands for circulation and the identification of internal bleeding, whether this is in the chest, the abdomen (for example from a ruptured spleen or liver damage) or from a fractured pelvis. Diagnosis of internal bleeding is difficult and requires experience; imaging of the body cavities is essential. Bleeding from broken thigh bones (femurs) can occasionally be severe enough to endanger life. The immediate treatment of internal bleeding is replacement of the lost blood. Historically this was usually with various salt solutions, but blood products are now usually used. Fractured long bones are splinted – femurs with versions of Thomas' splint, still a vital part of modern trauma management. We now know that Thomas' splint lowers mortality by reducing bleeding from broken bones, reducing the risk of fat embolism and preventing damage to local structures by the movement of ragged broken bone ends. It also dramatically reduces the patient's pain. Although some internal bleeding will stop in time, in many cases urgent surgery will be required. Generally, it takes longer to bleed to death internally than to die from a chest injury or blocked airway, hence its place in the ABCDE sequence.

"D" stands for disability, an initial assessment of brain and nerve function. This may not be necessary if the patient is talking coherently, but consists of an assessment of the pupils and how responsive the patient is: are they alert, or do they respond only to voice or pain? Are they unresponsive? Large pupils might suggest brain swelling, small pupils overdose with an opiate such as morphine or heroin. Unequal pupil sizes are an indicator of bleeding within the skull causing pressure on the nerves to the eye. An alternative assessment method is the Glasgow Coma Score, a more complex process which assesses speech, eye and limb movements. The Glasgow Coma Score is so widely accepted that even doctors in Edinburgh use it.

The final element of Styner's system is "E" (exposure). This is simply a head-to-toe examination of the patient to ensure that no other injury has been missed. As any life-threatening injury is identified, its treatment begins at once.

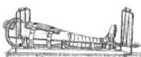

By the time "E" is reached, clinicians should have a good idea what the patient's life-threatening injuries are and have taken immediate steps to manage them. Many of these steps are simple, but require experience to recognise the need for them and skill to coordinate them in the most appropriate order and without avoidable delay. This is the role of the trauma team leader, pioneered at the BAH and now in use at all major trauma centres. The team leader must also make decisions in consultation with his colleagues regarding the need for general anaesthesia, opinions from other specialties, timing of scanning (usually head-to-toe CT scans), the need for blood transfusion and the timing and sequence of surgery. Managing the competing demands of different specialists can be challenging.

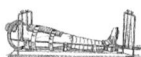

A major current textbook of trauma management in English practice states "*trauma victims do not, in a sense, die from trauma, but from the effects of trauma*". This might seem a philosophical point, but it highlights an essential truth of managing the critically injured. All the causes of death which are described in this chapter ultimately lead to one thing: the tissues and organs of the body do not receive enough oxygen. This may be because oxygen is not reaching the lungs, the lungs are not transferring oxygen to the blood or the blood is not carrying enough oxygen to the organs and tissues, either because there is not enough oxygen available or because there is not enough blood to carry it, or because the heart is pumping inadequately. As a result, the body becomes acidic (the medical term is acidotic). The cells of the human body are designed to function within a narrow range of parameters. Too acidotic and the blood clots less well, enzymes function less effectively or not at all. Specialist cells cease to function and ultimately break down. The mechanisms which maintain a stable and delicate internal environment begin to fail. Unchecked, death will surely follow.

The aim of treatment must therefore be to stop and reverse this process. This can be achieved by administering high concentrations of oxygen, providing a patent airway, ensuring the lungs function normally, replacing lost blood or supporting the pumping mechanism of the heart using drugs.

Second Interlude

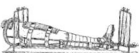

Some injuries are self-evidently immediately fatal. Amongst the others, even today there are injuries which are highly likely to be deadly with or without treatment, but these are becoming fewer, especially with rapid access to advanced medical care at the scene of the injury. Analytical methods allow the prediction of mortality rates for any given injury. Patients who, statistically, *should* not have survived, but do, are known as unexpected survivors and the number of these patients is a good measure of the effectiveness of any integrated trauma care system. As we will see in the next chapter, the BAH would play a pioneering role in the provision of expert assistance at the scene and lay the foundations for today's near-ubiquitous pre-hospital care provision. Bleeding from traumatic amputation can be rapidly controlled, stab wounds to the heart can be sutured after opening the chest, lacerations to abdominal organs can be managed with the rapid administration of blood. Even those who have suffered a cardiac arrest can sometimes be resuscitated. In all these cases, treatment must be started as soon as possible: these are time critical injuries and trauma care must be organised to treat them expeditiously. Unfortunately, head injuries, or more appropriately brain injuries, remain difficult to treat and are associated with a high mortality. Because the skull cannot expand, brain swelling leads to increased pressure and eventually brain cell death which is irreversible. Expert anaesthesia and sedation can do a great deal to prevent brain swelling, neurosurgeons can remove a flap of skull to allow the brain to expand. Despite this, severe brain injury retains its ability to kill, and when it doesn't, the effects on quality of life can be devastating because damaged brain tissue does not recover. We also now know that tiny changes in brain structure which are not visible on normal scans can result in alterations in behaviour and function which make return to normal life challenging.

Unfortunately, the trauma itself is not the only process which can result in death. It might be expected that the ability of blood to clot would be enhanced following trauma. In fact, blood clots less well after trauma and this in turn requires treatment with different elements of whole blood, including platelets and clotting factors. Platelets are the smallest human blood cells that congregate at the scene of bleeding, stick together and help to control haemorrhage; clotting factors circulate in the blood and in response to bleeding initiate blood clotting. Unfortunately, as bleeding continues, both may be used up and require replacement. Trauma also results in a generalised inflammatory response, which requires careful monitoring and management and risks damaging other tissues: organ failure may follow and require replacement therapy. Almost inevitably, many trauma victims become cold, either because they have been trapped in a vehicle, found at the bottom of a cliff, or unwisely undressed by medical staff and allowed to cool. We now know that becoming cold further reduces the ability of blood to clot, exacerbating bleeding and increasing mortality.

As we have already seen, when large bones break, they can release fat into the bloodstream which can travel to block veins, causing death of tissues due to the blockage and lack of blood supply. Although post-traumatic infection is no longer the killer it once was, it remains a significant problem. Once fractures become infected, eradication of the bacteria can be challenging and can seriously delay recovery. Patients who spend a long period of time in bed, and especially if they are in intensive care, are at risk of pneumonia. Prolonged bed rest is a risk factor for deep venous thrombosis and pulmonary embolism which can also be fatal.

It can be seen that to achieve the best outcomes for the critically injured, expert specialist care must be available as soon as possible after injury and ideally at the scene of the accident. In addition, such care must be multidisciplinary, carefully coordinated and not distracted by the injuries themselves, but guided by the effects of the trauma on the body's organs and systems. This is the Accident Hospital's legacy.

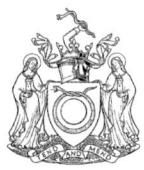

Chapter 5

Surgery on Wheels and in the Air

WILLIAM GISSANE NEVER considered the care of the injured to begin or end at the hospital door. Almost inevitably the Accident Hospital and its staff would play a major role in the development of the modern speciality of pre-hospital care, especially under the leadership of Keith Porter (later Professor Sir Keith Porter). As early as 1941, when the War looked like it might still be lost, and in response to a request from Gissane, the Austin Motor Company offered to present the hospital with a mobile surgical unit or MSU. This was a further example of the close working relationship between Gissane's team and Midland industry, especially the motor industry which accounted for 60% of the UK's total car production into the 1970s. Due to limitations on staff numbers because of the priorities of global war, the vehicle was not actually presented until 1947. It was agreed that a team would be provided consisting of a senior surgeon, assistant surgeon, anaesthetist and nurse. The Birmingham Hospitals Contributory Association undertook to maintain and garage the vehicle.

Now is a good time to introduce the immaculately dressed and mustachioed Peter London, known to all as "PSL" but prone to introducing himself as "London, Birmingham". London was born in Chile and came to Birmingham in 1948 after national Service in the RAF. As well as writing *A practical guide to the care of the injured* which became the bible for all junior surgeons with an interest in trauma and its management, he was also a regular crew leader on the MSU and in 1951 was called out to retrieve a man whose leg had been crushed under a tank. When he arrived, the tank was found to be unstable and at risk of collapsing on the rescuers. For this rescue he was awarded an MBE,

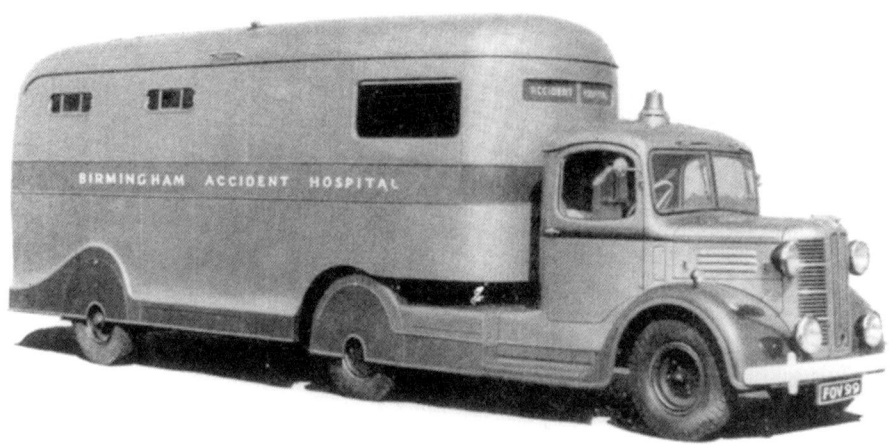

The mobile surgical unit.

in the words of the London Gazette: *"Dr London was in charge of the Mobile Surgical Unit which was summoned and on his arrival he immediately went to the trapped man and commenced anti-shock treatment. In order to release the man, hawsers were fixed to the tank which was then slowly raised from the wall on which it was resting. To prevent further injury to the man, Dr London jumped into the cavity between the wall and the still-moving tank so that he could support him. The Doctor was fully aware of the danger that the tank might fall back on him during the lifting operations, but without regard for his own safety he remained with the injured man until the latter had been released and removed to hospital."*

Peter London was internationally respected as a surgeon and advocate for the injured and like so many others, entered his surgical career after military service. Tragically, in 1977, his eldest son, Nick, fell during military training in the Brecon Beacons in Wales, rupturing his kidney. The emergency staff in the local hospital missed the diagnosis and he bled to death. London was told of his son's death whilst presenting a lecture, but in typical style went on to complete it. Peter London led team three which had an almost military atmosphere; many of the registrars were on secondment from the Army. One of London's consultant colleagues was Tom Matherson, an avid pipe smoker who on one occasion in outpatients set his white coat on fire when he failed to extinguish his pipe effectively.

The intention behind the mobile surgical unit was to take the treatment of the critically injured to the accident scene. Early intervention in trauma is now accepted as the key to any effective trauma service and the justification for our air ambulance services and pre-hospital care schemes. In the 1940s it was radical in the extreme. Indeed, in the decades to come, there would be years of agonised debate within the

5. Surgery on Wheels and in the Air

medical profession regarding the need for pre-hospital medicine at all. Arguments about the value of doctors providing care before arrival in hospital would continue with acrimony into the twenty-first century. Now pre-hospital medicine is a speciality in its own right with its own consultants and its own professional qualifications. As we have seen, many of the life-threatening problems that follow trauma can be managed relatively easily, but only if appropriately skilled personnel are available in good time: this is the basis for medical pre-hospital care. Lives are now saved on a daily basis by the provision of expert medical care at the scene of an accident and the mobile surgical unit was, as we shall see, one of the key steps on the way, not because it established a model for future practice, but because it was the first step in a culture change which led to the acceptance of pre-hospital medical provision as a concept.

Given its size, the MSU must have been a striking sight trundling around Birmingham, but it was hardly nippy and its obvious defect was the fact that the casualty tended to get to the BAH before the MSU got to the patient. On occasion, however, when the patient was trapped, it must have appeared to the patient as a vision of safety. It was with these patients where the presence of a skilled surgeon able to release the patient from their predicament really made a difference. The MSU also attended incidents in areas covered only by small district general hospitals, when it

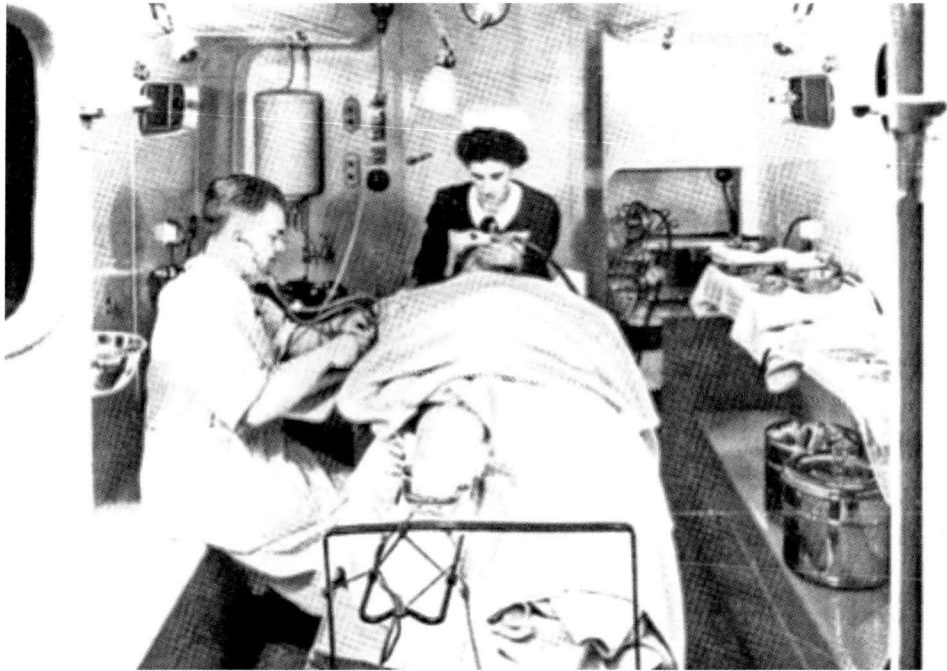

Inside the mobile surgical unit.

also occasionally carried out life-saving surgery. On one occasion a young woman's life was saved by a blood transfusion following a miscarriage. The commonest cause for a call-out to a child was burns resulting from their clothes catching fire.

Ultimately, the mobile surgical unit was a failure. It was only infrequently used, treating seven patients in its first year of operation and only 136 by the time it was taken out of service in 1954. Around half the incidents were industrial accidents, a quarter road traffic accidents and a further quarter accidents in the home. One patient was injured shooting rabbits and the unit also attended an aeroplane crash. The MSU was a noble attempt to take treatment to the scene of an accident and although it was short-lived, it would lead eventually to radical changes in the immediate management of the critically injured.

Articulated and much larger than a modern ambulance, the MSU had two main sections, both temperature controlled, one containing an operating table with space for stretchers on either side, the other equipment and a writing desk. The equipment was remarkably comprehensive for the time and included drugs, Thomas' famous splints, dressings, intravenous fluids, tourniquets, ice for preserving body parts and, remarkably, blood. Blood would not be routinely available in the pre-hospital environment until the twenty-first century after extensive experience in Afghanistan. When the MSU was called out, the house surgeon on call was sent to collect the blood from the refrigerator in the laboratories and put it in the ice box in the vehicle. At night, ice was collected from the refrigerator in the main kitchen and used to keep the bottles of blood cold (at this time blood was supplied in glass bottles which could produce dramatic consequences when one was dropped). When the ambulance was called out during the daytime these duties were carried out by the sister in charge of the casualty operating theatre. Arrangements were in place to return the blood to the blood bank if it wasn't used. Sterilising facilities were also available on the vehicle, although probably never used, and the other equipment included amputation kits and all the equipment for administering a general anaesthetic – not to mention such mundane but vital articles as oxygen, bed pans and urinals. As well as bringing skilled medical and nursing care to the scene of the accident, the MSU also provided a safe and effective environment for the transfer of the injured back to the Accident Hospital.

The true significance of the Mobile Surgical Unit was not in the relatively small number of patients it treated, but in indicating a direction of travel which would ultimately lead to today's universal provision of skilled and advanced pre-hospital care as part of an integrated care network. At a time when taking the doctor to the accident was unheard of, it demonstrated both that skilled medical care could be taken to the scene of an accident and that such interventions made a significant difference to the outcome for individual patients.

5. Surgery on Wheels and in the Air

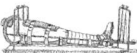

It is hard to imagine now, but before 1989 there was very little provision of advanced clinical support to ambulance personnel; indeed, the profession of paramedic itself was still new. Where doctors provided care at the scene of accidents or other emergencies, it was usually provided by general practitioners based in their own practice areas and often required them to leave a busy surgery to attend to the needs of an accident victim or desperately sick patient. Pre-hospital care in Britain is built on the foundations of a generation of general practitioners determined to offer the best possible care they could, at no charge, to the injured in the areas in which they practiced. It is ironic, therefore, but perhaps inevitable, that the majority of pre-hospital care, and especially that which is carried out by helicopter, is now implemented by doctors in hospital specialties. Despite this, in the mostly rural and remote areas, the provision of such care remains largely in the hands of family doctors, augmented as appropriate by helicopter medical services. In December 1989 a series of ambulance strikes began and some services were taken over by the Armed Forces and the police. Keith Porter, then newly appointed to the Accident Hospital, and who defined major trauma as *"when the patient arrives at hospital in more than one ambulance"*, identified a number of cases where lack of expert care had had a negative effect on the patient's outcome. These included a lady with a spinal injury who became paralysed as a result of inappropriate handling and a haemorrhaging patient whose bleeding was not adequately controlled. As a result of these concerns and in association with the Chief Officer of West Midlands Ambulance Service, a mobile medical response team based at the Accident Hospital was established. The team was voluntary and included doctors from consultants to registrars and nurses of all levels of seniority. As a result, almost 800 calls were undertaken with vehicles and equipment provided by West Midlands Ambulance Service responding, unusually, to a mixture of trauma and medical cases including cardiac arrests.

After the strike came to an end, the new voluntary service was continued and formally established in 1990 as the Central Accident Resuscitation Emergency (CARE) Team. In its early years, the CARE Team would provide expert care every Friday and Saturday night from 18.00 to 02.00, offering advanced airway care, intravenous access and advanced pain relief. The team travelled from incident to incident in a vehicle driven by a member of the West Midlands Ambulance Service and consisted of a doctor and a nurse, both providing their services free of charge. Breaks were taken in ambulance stations or laybys and there was a remarkable sense of camaraderie with the other emergency services.

The CARE Team, which continues to aid the sick and injured of the West Midlands, now on a daily basis, was one of the first of the pre-hospital care providers which now cover the whole of the country and form a key component, as we shall see, of modern integrated trauma networks. Clinicians who cut their teeth in accident scene care in the CARE Team have gone on to play important roles in the development of pre-hospital care as a speciality and in bringing advanced care to the home or the roadside.

It was only a small step from the land based CARE Team response car to delivering care by air. The Midlands Air Ambulance flew on its first mission in 1990. As with the CARE Team, the medical crew of the first callout carrying a doctor was Keith Porter. The first patient, a coach driver injured in a road traffic collision (or road traffic accident as they were known at the time) was flown back to the Accident Hospital. Except on occasions when the nature of the incident or information about the patient's injuries suggested the need for a doctor, in its early days, the helicopter normally only carried a paramedic; medical advice was provided remotely by radio from a consultant at the hospital. In the early 1990s the helicopter brought a patient to the hospital on average twice a week. It is much busier nowadays, the air ambulance carries a senior doctor trained in pre-hospital emergency care and a critical care paramedic (a profession which didn't exist in the 1990s). The original base at RAF Cosford has now grown to three operating locations.

A number of staff of the Accident Hospital were also involved in various kinds of motorsport. Some acted in their professional capacity and some as marshals or members of dedicated rescue teams.

From the early 1980s the hospital also offered offer a rescue unit with a doctor and another medical unit as part of the emergency cover for what was then the Lombard RAC Rally, as well as for elements of the World Rally Championship. The rescue unit, which was equipped with tools to extract trapped competitors, also offered advanced first aid to competitors, spectators and officials if needed. In true "Acci" tradition, the medical units were kitted out with donations from several companies and for a number of years the local Mercedes dealership generously loaned two 4-wheel-drive 'G Wagons'. The ability of these vehicles to survive accidents, for example when one skidded on oil and hit a tree, turned out to be a selling point exploited by the company. Each unit was crewed by a doctor, nurse and driver or paramedic and allocated several stages of the race which took place in November across Wales, Northern England and on occasion southern Scotland. Eventually, changes in the organisation of the race meant that the hospital's resources were no longer needed, although many individuals continued their personal commitment to providing cover at motor racing and other sporting events. It is very likely that this cover was one of the first, if not the first example of expert medical care being made available to a sporting event.

5. Surgery on Wheels and in the Air

In retrospect, the involvement of Accident Hospital staff in a wide range of trauma care provision was indicative of the fact that, as in so much of the Health Service, being a healthcare professional was not just a job, it was a way of life, as part of which demands on staff or at least expectations which would now be considered completely unacceptable, were routine, expected and (generally) enjoyed. Consultants in particular were expected to undertake unpaid work, but many staff from all professions and specialties worked without reward or recognition considerably beyond the hours for which they were paid.

Staff from the BAH played a leading role in breaking down the concept that advanced medical care to the seriously injured began at the door of the emergency department. The skilled and experienced doctors, nurses and paramedics who attend such scenes today are their heirs and bear witness to Gissane's vision of trauma care from point of injury to rehabilitation.

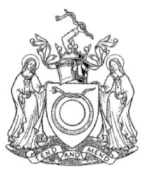

Third Interlude

21st November 1974

IN THE EARLY evening of Thursday 21st November, central Birmingham was going about its usual midweek business. The shops were closed, the night darkening, the streets full of those looking to enjoy a night "in town". The Mulberry Bush and Tavern in the Town pubs were crowded with punters enjoying a drink after work or looking forward to a night of more serious indulgence. Curry houses were then, as now, an essential component of a Birmingham night out, Mitchells and Butlers the beer of choice for a night on the lash.

Ten days earlier there had been a number of small explosions, one of which was in the iconic 25 storey Rotunda office block on New Street, but there had been no serious injuries. At about 8.30pm on the 21st, the night was torn apart by the sounds of two massive explosions only ten minutes apart. The first explosion was in the Mulberry Bush on the ground floor of the Rotunda office block; the second bomb exploded nearby in the underground Tavern in the Town, only a few hundred yards along New Street. The bombs had been concealed in briefcases or duffel bags. The explosion at the Tavern in the Town blew several victims through a brick wall. Rescue attempts were hampered by the destruction of the stairway from street level and the presence of electric cabling exposed by the blast. A passing bus was also destroyed.

21 people died, most at the scenes, some in hospital and more than 200 were injured, the majority were young people on an enjoyable night out. Of the ten people who died in the Mulberry explosion, two had simply been walking past when the bomb detonated. Many of the victims suffered traumatic amputations. The pattern of injuries

Third Interlude

reflected those seen in countless terrorist bombings before and since. Bombs are, for very good reason, the terrorist's weapon of choice. Apart from anything else they can be left to detonate long after the bomber has left the scene, or detonated remotely. Thus the perpetrator can ensure that others die for his cause without risk to himself. It is also in the nature of bombs that the injuries they inflict are mutilating and horrific; victims are hit by bits of metal, body parts and debris, bodies are shattered and limbs torn away. The choice of location means that many of the victims are likely to know each other in social or family groups, dramatically increasing the psychological effects of the incident. Bombs are truly a weapon of terror and their injuries require specialist and expert care. As we shall see, Birmingham will in due course become the country's leading centre for the management of such injuries, albeit those inflicted thousands of miles away by equally cowardly perpetrators in Afghanistan and Iraq.

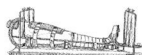

The Birmingham Pub Bombings, as they came to be called, were the deadliest attacks in the United Kingdom between the end of the Second World War and those of 7th July 2005 in London. Police had attempted to clear both pubs after a man with an Irish accent telephoned the *Birmingham Post* newspaper with a warning and recognised password, but the bombs detonated only 12 minutes after the call. It was

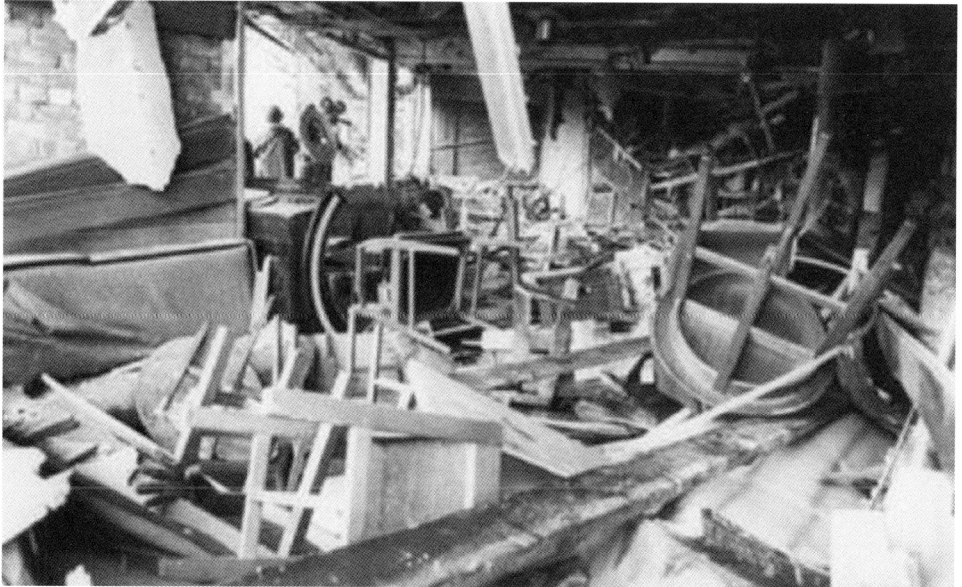

The Mulberry Bush pub – after the explosion.

later alleged that the call was delayed because the public telephone box which the bomber intended to use had been vandalised and precious minutes were lost whilst the bomber found another one: as a result, evacuation of the premises was impossible. A third bomb had been planted on the Hagley Road, just outside the city centre. Although the detonator of this device activated when a policeman prodded the plastic bag in which it had been left with his truncheon, fortunately the bomb itself did not explode. It was later destroyed by a bomb disposal team.

After the second explosion, every pub and office in the city centre was evacuated by the police and the nearby City Hotel was established as a first aid post. As each survivor was extricated from the scene, they were evacuated on makeshift stretchers made from tables and doors.

The Irish Republican Army (IRA) was immediately identified by the Security Services as the most likely perpetrators of the bombings, which would become infamous for the carnage they caused, and, later, for the miscarriage of justice which resulted from the conviction of those not responsible for the atrocity.

The IRA did not admit responsibility for the attacks at the time (despite the use of an accepted IRA codeword) and have not done so since, despite calls for them to do so.

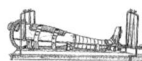

Today, the response to any incident of this kind is carefully structured with pre-arranged levels of command and pre-allotted tasks for each of the emergency services. Almost 50 years ago, lessons were still being learnt from a series of terrorist atrocities in Northern Ireland and although such incidents were becoming more common on the United Kingdom mainland, significant numbers of casualties were rare and on the scale of the Birmingham bombings unprecedented. Police, the fire brigade and ambulance crews attended the scene immediately, but it would be almost 50 minutes before a formal declaration of a major incident was made.

Birmingham's taxi drivers helped ferry the injured to the Accident and General hospitals. The cabbies also assisted by taking home those who had declined hospital treatment and those who had been discharged after hospital treatment. No payment was accepted by the drivers. Casualties also arrived by private car and ambulance as well as on foot, the Accident Hospital being only a mile from the scene of the bombings. Some also walked to the General Hospital which was somewhat closer to the scenes. The Accident Hospital alone would receive 198 casualties on the day of the incident and about 100 of these, who were the walking wounded, were carried by the cabbies from the New Street Station rank. Within an hour of the bombs going off 100 casualties arrived. By the time the immediate incident was over, the hospital had

Third Interlude

received 217 victims. Like all terrorist incidents, the bombings would, in time, leave a long tail of investigations, wound dressings, further surgery and rehabilitation which would keep the hospital's staff busy for months.

As the patients arrived, staff began attending hospital from home having seen the first reports of the bombs on television. The casualty theatre and the plaster theatre became ordinary operating theatres and casualties were brought to the Major Incident Unit until it was full, after which they were received in casualty. The medical records department immediately began compiling patient information for the police. This information was handed over in person at Steelhouse Lane Police Station as the police radio system had failed and was no longer functioning. Prior to the pub bombings, an Army Captain had been attempting to diffuse a bomb in Edgbaston close to a girl's school. Tragically the device had been booby trapped and detonated during the attempt to defuse it. The officer survived for ten days before dying of his injuries at the Accident Hospital. As a consequence, throughout this time and during the response to the pub bombings, Special Branch personnel toured the hospital as a security measure. They were both heavily armed and heavy footed, so much so that complaints were made that they were keeping patients awake through the night. As the event progressed patients would require police protection from intrusive reporters. Later, and in true BAH tradition, the hospital bar would be kept open by the steward and would only close at 4.00am, providing a place of relative refuge for staff and police officers alike. Throughout the incident, the hospital's catering staff provided a continuous supply of free bacon sandwiches.

In a minor stroke of luck, the bombs detonated around 8.30pm which was close to the handover time of the hospital's day and night shifts, and as a result many of the day staff were still in the hospital and were able to help. There were also four staff social get-togethers in progress within walking distance, allowing nurses, blood technicians, radiographers and other staff (both past and present) to attend within a few minutes. Those at home responded to early bulletins on the nine o'clock news only minutes after the bombs went off.

Inevitably at first, the sheer number of wounded overwhelmed the staff on duty and the immediately available facilities. Unsurprisingly, although staff had years of experience dealing with trauma, they had not had to cope with the typical injuries associated with terrorist bombs. As increasing numbers of off-duty staff started arriving to assist, the situation came more under control. Members of the St John Ambulance Brigade turned out, and some off-duty police officers, who were in the city centre arrived with wounded members of the public, and stayed to help. Eventually the hospital would receive so many calls from nurses offering to help that an individual had to be allocated to answer them. As is so often the case in very challenging circumstances, morale in the hospital was very high.

Each patient was searched by a nurse looking for identification and every patient was photographed and given a photographic identity number. Inevitably some patients were severely mutilated and many were covered in dirt, debris, dust and blood. In the days that followed, the hospital photographers would be called upon to take photographs of the surviving victims and also at the post-mortems.

Because the bombs had gone off in pubs, many of the victims were known to each other, their innocent social evening shattered by terrorism. Separating casualties according to their clinical need was therefore often difficult and charged with emotion. Gradually, however, as the hours passed, the situation became one of organisation and quiet determination to do the best for so many injured victims. Most patients passed from casualty to the operating theatres and then to the Major Injuries Unit or wards; inevitably, and tragically, some died and were taken in the first instance to the hospital mortuary before eventually being transferred to the nearby Coroner's Mortuary. Photographs were taken of the dead to record their identification and the nature of their injuries.

Outside the hospital, where relative calm reigned, the city centre was gridlocked, the silence shattered by multiple alarms set of by the blasts. The streets surrounding the bomb sites were full of broken glass and debris, emergency vehicles and personnel worked at considerable risk to themselves given the possibility of a secondary device. Morale amongst the responders and rescuers remained high with the sense of camaraderie that so often occurs in those responding to a critical incident.

In the days that followed, both the home secretary Roy Jenkins and the Prime Minister Harold Macmillan would visit the hospital to speak to the victims and to thank the staff. In due course, HM the Queen would invite staff from the hospital to a thank you private reception.

The explosions coincided with the return to Ireland of the body of James McDade, an IRA terrorist who had been killed in Coventry the previous week when the bomb he was planting blew up prematurely. The prime suspects for the Birmingham Bombings had gone to school with McDade and came to police attention as they went to Ireland for his funeral. They were arrested at Fishguard on return to the UK and subsequent tests on their hands for explosive residue were positive. However, it was later realised that the same positive results were possible from exposure to new playing cards or British Rail polish used on carriage tables. The fact that British Rail had polish for their tables in 1974 may be a surprise to anyone who remembers using trains in the 1970s. Nevertheless, in 1975, six men were found guilty of carrying out the bombings. Eventually becoming known as the Birmingham Six, they were released in 1991 after 16 years in prison, when their convictions were overturned by the Court of Appeal. Those really responsible for the Birmingham Pub Bombings have never been brought to justice.

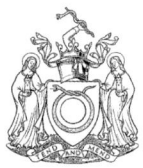

Chapter 6

Still Innovating

AS THE 1960s progressed and turned into the 1970s, the hospital, still unique in its provision of specialist trauma care, lost none of its appetite for innovation. It continued to be a pioneer of many of the techniques commonly used in the modern management of the victims of trauma. A particular development popularised at the BAH was the use of tracheostomy, making a hole in the front of a patient's neck for a tube through which they could be effectively ventilated. Tracheostomy also allowed secretions to be removed from the lungs by suction and was a significant breakthrough, especially in the management of patients with severe head injuries and all those who needed prolonged ventilation. Chest infections became fewer and many patients no longer needed to be managed on the Major Injuries Unit, but could be managed on a special tracheostomy ward, one of the forerunners of today's high dependency units. Unfortunately, the initiative was not at first a success. The high levels of humidity needed to ensure that lung secretions were kept moist and could be suctioned away paradoxically led to an unacceptably high level of infections and, remarkably, there were complaints from staff that the moisture levels were causing the bee hive hair-dos so popular at the time to collapse! The ward, which can't have been a particularly pleasant place in which either to be ill, or to work, was closed after two years. The technique, however, went on to become a mainstay of modern intensive care medicine.

The ability to take images of injuries and the complexity of potential investigations developed throughout the lifetime of the hospital, although many of the cutting-edge technologies of 50 years ago have now been replaced by much less invasive investigations. From the beginning a consultant surgeon was involved in the management of every patient. This meant that the most appropriate investigations could be ordered, that they were performed without delay and that the results could be fed back to the clinical team as a matter of urgency. For decades after the hospital opened, X-ray films (or "radiographs", but never "X-rays" – *"you can't see X-rays dear boy, never mind hold them!"*) were developed using a wet chemical technique, a method now lost with digital imaging. One of the jobs of the most junior member of the team was to provide the consultant with the appropriate film when requested. Unless an X-ray viewing box was taken on the ward round, images were viewed by holding them up to the light or on occasion sticking them to a convenient window with a dab of spit. Only in the last few years before the hospital closed was the process automated and the dark room technician no longer required.

When the Accident Hospital's blood transfusion service was established in 1952, it was the first hospital to have one. From then on emergency blood transfusion was available 24 hours a day. Like many of the hospital's initiatives, the service was improvised and depended on the commitment of a small number of staff; in this case seven members of staff from the hospital laboratories, MRC Industrial Injuries and Burns Units who had undertaken a course of instruction from Dr Sevitt.

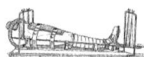

The Road Injuries Research Group had been founded by William Gissane and John Bull in 1960 at the suggestion of Dr Donald Stewart, chief medical officer of the Austin Motor Company and member of the governing body of the AA. The hospital provided accommodation and the AA paid for a secretary for the first ten years after which the MRC took over. Until this time, the majority of cars on British roads were essentially tin boxes with wheels – safety being a very minor consideration. The secretary was Miss Barbara Roberts who collated the details of all the fatal road accidents around Birmingham in 1960. Her data would lead to recommendations for design improvements to cars and lorries. We have already seen some of the changes in vehicle design introduced as a result of the group's activities, but it also recommended combining the diagonal seat belt (favoured by the Swedes but risking strangulation if there was a side impact accident) and the lap belt (favoured by the Americans) to produce the seat belts still in general use today. One area of study was of fatalities on the new M1 motorway, work which led to the introduction of collapsible, telescopic steering columns. Professor Gissane (he was made the United Kingdom's first professor of accident surgery in 1961) was asked to assist Rover designers to help make

6. Still Innovating

a much safer car. He contributed the concepts of the passenger "safety zone", the "crumple zone", and a number of other initiatives, including minimum tyre standards and the removal of elements from the front of a car capable of becoming detached or inflicting unnecessary injury in the event of an impact.

In 1961 The Accident Service Review Committee report (the Platt Report) resulted in the creation of five major accident and emergency departments in and around Birmingham thus reducing the BAH's caseload. The 1972 Scott Review led to the change from orthopaedic surgeons being in charge of the casualty department and paved the way for the development of the speciality of emergency medicine. Although this was undoubtedly a huge step forward for patients, it would, in the long term, be a contributing factor in the closure of the Accident Hospital which, uniquely, and reasonably given its specialist practice in trauma, maintained the old orthopaedic-led model.

Other initiatives by clinicians at the BAH were less dramatic in their immediate impact, but each made a difference to the care of the injured. Perhaps the most important of these was the introduction of the tangential excision of burnt skin. This is a technique by which very thin slices of skin are taken for use as skin grafts and placed on areas of skin loss elsewhere. The technique, which is a staple of current surgical practice and has unquestionably saved many lives, is not dissimilar to using an old-fashioned potato peeler, but with more blood. The burns team would also be amongst the first to culture skin cells in the laboratory.

That the victims of trauma, especially if they are immobilised or confined to bed, are at risk of blood clots, which can be fatal, has already been seen. Unfortunately, prevention of this problem still does not always receive the attention it deserves. This may be because the victims of trauma are very often young and do not fall into the categories of patients generally accepted to be at risk of clotting disorders, or simply that the risk is forgotten amongst multiple other claims on clinicians' time in the early stages of resuscitation of the desperately injured. Blood clots most commonly form in the veins of the leg as deep venous thromboses (often called DVTs) and if they break up may travel through the bloodstream to the lungs, causing the blockage of blood vessels (embolisation) which can be fatal. Dr Sevitt at the BAH was a pioneer in the use of anticoagulants to prevent clotting. To scepticism from colleagues, he used warfarin, developed as a highly effective rat poison, to dramatically reduce the number of thromboses and emboli in trauma patients. Warfarin remains a mainstay of anticoagulation to this day.

The scientists weren't the only innovators as the hospital continued to push the boundaries of trauma care. One of the surgeons, J.H. Hicks, was a pioneer of the use of metal plates to stabilise fractures and encourage healing, designing a perforated plate which was placed across a fracture and secured in place with screws.

Developments of Hicks' plate remain essential tools in modern orthopaedics. Hicks had seen service as a ship's surgeon during World War II before his appointment the BAH and was also a botanist of distinction who joined an expedition to Bhutan and had two plants named after him.

Undoubtedly the greatest breakthrough in trauma management in the twenty-first century has been the recognition and acceptance that the best treatment for the trauma victim who has lost blood is administration of blood, or more usually blood products. As a bald statement of fact, this seems so obvious that it is difficult to believe that any other approach was ever considered. In fact, until very recently much time, effort and money were invested in attempts to determine precisely which *other* fluid was most appropriate for administration to trauma victims. Other areas of research interest included methods of administration. Possibilities seriously considered included intravenous, subcutaneous (under the skin) and rectal (up the bottom) fluids. It should also be remembered that until relatively recently, trauma was treated by removing blood ("blood-letting") with predictably catastrophic results. For most of the twentieth century, the standard fluids given to trauma patients were normal saline (salt water at a similar concentration to human blood) and Hartmann's solution (a slightly more complex salt solution named after its inventor). Blood was seen as an additional therapy to be used sparingly and only when experience in Afghanistan proved beyond doubt that the best replacement fluid was blood (or its components) did practice in the majority of centres change. Until then long-standing practice dictated that blood be given in "doses" of two or four pints, irrespective of the amount of blood lost. The first small step on the road to modern fluid therapy occurred at the BAH when Ruscoe Clarke, founder of the MIU, not only changed practice by insisting that the amount of blood administered reflected closely an estimate of the amount of blood lost, but insisted that potentially very large volumes of blood were administered if the patient needed them. Thus Clarke was one of the first to identify the fact that early transfusion of the correct volume of whole blood appeared to lead to the best chance of quick and full recovery from serious injury. He also coined the term "the golden 20 minutes" to refer to the optimal time after injury for resuscitating a victim of trauma. This concept would later become the "golden hour" and drove an often-lacking sense of urgency in resuscitating the trauma patient. One of the pioneers of tracheostomy, Clarke's popularising of this technique would in turn lead to developments in medical drains, tubes, filters and methods of humidifying inhaled gases. During the London Blitz Ruscoe Clarke had worked in shock research as well as later serving abroad with RAMC. Like many of his contemporaries, Clarke brought his extensive military experience to Birmingham to the immense benefit of his patients. He joined the Accident Hospital team in 1947 where his particular interest was, as we have seen, shock, the subject of his important work on blood transfusion. Clarke became Secretary of the Institute of Accident Surgery in 1951 and, unlike the majority of his contemporaries, was a committed communist and an active member of the British Peace Committee. In 1947 during the run-up to the formation of the National Health Service, his wife recalled: *"Ruscoe came home white and shaking after a meeting at Birmingham Town Hall in 1947... All the doctors in Birmingham were opposing the very concept of a National Health Service and supporting the retention of private practice. Ruscoe was the only doctor to speak in favour of the NHS and abolition of private patients."*

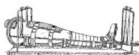

These developments in trauma management occurred against a background of busy clinical practice. Operating theatres were available, and used, 24 hours a day. Modern practice restricts night-time operating, but until the hospital closed, life-saving surgery would routinely be followed in the middle of the night by semi-urgent surgery, such as the repair of fractures or reduction of dislocations. The BAH's operating theatres were large enough to allow more than one patient to be operated on in each theatre if the capacity was required. At the time the hospital closed, its main operating theatres employed more than 30 staff, supported by a busy instrument curator's department which was also responsible for providing dressings, appliances, splints and surgical implants. Much minor surgery continued to be performed in the three casualty theatres which were separately staffed. For generations of Birmingham medical students stitching minor wounds in these theatres was their introduction to real patients. For many years the curator's department was under the supervision and eagle eye of Bill Cater. Trained as a nurse, Cater saw war service in Europe and Africa where he developed his talents for inventing novel but effective surgical appliances. He joined the BAH in 1947 and was soon recognised as being able to "make or mend anything". He was also an early pioneer of the role of the operating theatre practitioner, now ubiquitous in operating theatres. Improvisation was not confined to the instrument curator's department, however. Dr Colin Thomas, director of the Major Injuries Unit (MIU), was renowned for making intensive care equipment from jubilee clips and other "found objects". His constructions included an improvised machine to provide the then novel, but now universally accepted capability of non-invasive ventilation (ventilation via a face mask rather than a tube in the windpipe). At the time, no machine was commercially available. Another example of this improvisational approach was the manufacture of an oxygen hood out of a plastic bucket with oxygen tubing inserted through a hole burned in its bottom with a cigarette lighter and an improvised valve based on the bucket's handle. This was used to provide oxygen for an infant suffering from smoke inhalation when no other equipment was available. Thomas' approach to the medical management of patients was equally imaginative and he was a pioneer in introducing new ventilation techniques in the critically injured.

Even as staff struggled to accept that the BAH was likely to close, teaching and research remained a priority. Mr Kaya Emin Alpar, an eminent trauma surgeon of Turkish extraction and pioneer of postgraduate trauma education, established a master's degree at Birmingham University. It was said of him that *"he pioneered a course in surgery of trauma that became world renowned"*. His approach, in classic Accident Hospital style, was that the trauma surgeon must be a generalist because trauma does not observe anatomical boundaries. Prof Graham Ayliffe was a medical microbiologist widely regarded nationally and internationally as the founder of infection prevention and control. After service in the Royal Navy, he qualified in medicine and joined the Hospital Infection Research Laboratory at the BAH in 1964. He was instrumental in founding the Infection Control Nurses Association in 1970 and for describing a widely used six step hand-washing technique that was later endorsed by the World Health Organisation. His best-known publication was *The Control of Hospital Infection – A Practical Handbook*. He later became director of the research laboratory where he carried out seminal work on the science underpinning infection prevention and control. His areas of research included hand hygiene and alcoholic hand disinfection, isolation wards, the emergence of antibiotic resistance, the role of disinfectants and the decontamination of equipment and the environment. In 1987 he helped found the International Federation for Infection Control in association with the World Health Organisation.

The focus of teaching was not solely on Birmingham. Mr Peter Bewes, born in Nairobi to missionary parents, was a general surgeon who worked in both Uganda and Tanzania, before joining the staff of the Birmingham Accident Hospital. He was a pioneer in developing surgical techniques and management approaches for clinicians in under-resourced countries for whom he wrote his acclaimed book *Surgery*. He was co-author of *Primary Surgery* which is still in print as a guide for surgeons where facilities are limited. Amongst his tips were the use of fishing line as surgical thread and of traction in the treatment of femoral fractures, a technique which had been replaced by surgical fixation in the First World but offered an effective cheap treatment method in less well-developed countries. After his retirement he returned to Uganda as chief surgeon to the government and worked to develop the country's medical system and especially its medical education. Graeme Dickson, last consultant anaesthetist to be appointed to the BAH, was part of a team sent from the Burns Unit to assist in a fire disaster in Jamshedpur in India in 1992 at the request of the Foreign and Commonwealth Office and Paul Levick, consultant burns and plastics surgeon, created the Bright Eyes charity for the provision of reconstructive surgery for war victims, predominantly children from Afghanistan, Pakistan and Lebanon. He operated on these patients in their home countries but also brought them back to the UK for surgery – all funded by the charity.

By the late 1970s, the BAH was treating 20,000 patients each year, of whom 5,000 were inpatients. Perhaps surprisingly almost 25% of patients still attended as the result of industrial accidents. More than 200 had sustained a domestic accident and only 6% attended as a result of a road traffic collision, although this figure was 18.9% amongst inpatients and vehicle accidents accounted for 30% of deaths. As closure approached, these numbers only increased; in 1989/90, 50,000 new casualty cases were seen as well as 35,000 outpatient attendances and there were 5,500 inpatients. That same year, the total cost of running the hospital was £8.3 million. This remarkable figure reflects the relatively small size of the hospital. At the time of closure it employed only 50 full-time medical staff, of whom only 11 were consultants, 253 nurses, 31 rehabilitation staff and around 250 staff in all the other departments. There were also small numbers of part-time medical staff in the smaller specialties, such as care of the elderly, chest surgery and ophthalmology and in the laboratory-based disciplines.

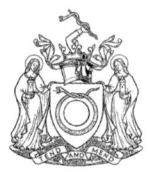

Chapter 7

The Head Injuries Club

HEAD INJURIES ARE common in both civilian and war trauma with potentially devastating long-term consequences for patients and their families. Recent combat experience has suggested that even mild head injuries may have significant long-term consequences which are often overlooked. Even today, with increasing recognition of the problem, follow up, support and rehabilitation for head-injured patients is often poor or non-existent. The increasing skill and knowledge of the staff at the Accident Hospital meant that ever-larger numbers of head-injured patients each year survived but many of them had severe and persisting problems. These included the inability to return to work, personality changes, communication problems, memory loss and impaired mental function. Conventional therapy seemed to be of limited use but there was a clear need to address the issue. Fortunately the early NHS allowed considerably greater latitude for individual initiative without the necessity for a needs analysis, attitude survey, SWAT analysis, multiple mission statements, or endless working parties and, as a consequence, it was relatively simple for Accident Hospital staff to identify the need and to establish a solution.

What the head-injured needed first of all was a sense of community with a chance to develop friendships with similarly afflicted patients in a supportive environment facilitated by expert staff (although the staff too were learning as the service developed). Given the attitude of the day to those with long-term health needs, the initial expectation of all but the clinicians involved was that only a minority of patients would ever be able to earn their own living independently. However, within a very short time, as a published report commented, significant numbers of patients were able to achieve a level of function sufficient for them to be able to earn their living independent of support. That they were, and continued to be, able to do so was very largely due to the efforts of an inspirational figure.

Jack Thackeray (not to be confused with the lugubrious songwriter Jake Thackray), like so many of the hospital's staff was an army veteran having served as an infantry soldier. He became a physical training sergeant instructor before leaving the Forces and settling as a youth leader in his home city of Leeds. After training as a remedial gymnast, Thackeray joined the BAH, taking responsibility for patients with severe head injuries. After a variety of jobs elsewhere, including Uganda, he returned to the BAH in the late 60s to transform the rehabilitation of head-injured patients in an unholy alliance with Miss Savage (the Head Occupational Therapist). Together they would achieve remarkable things.

"*Thackeray's behaviour with his patients, particularly in the Hospital's gymnasium, could easily have been mistaken for that of a bully, but a bully behaves as he does for his own disreputable satisfaction. What Thackeray recognised was the need to challenge and stretch his patients and thereby to try to replace in the injured brain patterns of perception and reaction that would become part of more purposeful and everyday activity.*" It would be interesting to compare Thackeray's approach with modern rehabilitation, of which we will hear more in due course. The writer goes on "*if his authoritative, no-nonsense insistence and persistence caused resentment in his patients that resentment fired their determination to 'show him', which may have been combined with less than complimentary thoughts. Whatever they may have felt at the time, none of his patients or their relatives could have been anything but admiringly grateful for what he enabled them to do.*"

Thackeray, like so many of his generation was not swayed by the need to be popular, but was motivated solely by the need to do his duty to those in his care. Injured patients were brought from the wards to the gym every day, even before they were able to stand. Thackeray invented an early walking frame using tubing from orthopaedic beds and later, patients would in their turn make similar frames from wood. He also designed a more complex system of harness, ropes and pulleys in a mobile frame which gave some mobility to those not yet ready to walk: three assistants, one on the arms, one the legs and one giving instructions, began the slow process of the patients' return to mobility. Thackeray's approach would eventually be followed by the expert rehabilitation teams managing the terribly injured service personnel returning from the wars in Iraq and Afghanistan.

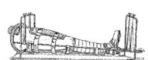

As the 1960s progressed staff at the BAH were presented with a new problem. Advances in medicine meant that patients were surviving what would once have been fatal head injuries. Many of those affected were young men from motorcycle accidents. The BAH pioneered the treatment of severe brain damage, by immediate tracheotomy or intubation – which saved lives, but increased the pool of patients with multiple disabilities. These patients naturally required more than the usual rehabilitation and inevitably these advances were not matched by the development of rehabilitation and community-based care. As a consequence, people with head injuries were being discharged into the care of their families with limited support or into inappropriate institutions. Rehabilitation being so well established at the BAH and in the hands of such devoted and determined staff, it was inevitable that the hospital would offer pioneering services to the head-injured.

The Head Injuries Club, founded in 1962 by Jack Thackeray, Peter London and Philip Lockhart the chief almoner (social worker), became a vital element in patient recovery. It was based on a similar facility Lockhart had encountered in London for stroke victims. Its mission was to *"provide opportunities for members to participate in group activities in order to help restore their confidence, promote mutual support and encouragement and to develop their potential, thereby assisting them to live as full a life as possible within the limits imposed by disability, and to help others in similar circumstances to do the same..."*

More than 100 people attended the opening meeting and subsequently enthusiasm was sustained as activities broadened and expanded. Thackeray especially was a big presence on Monday evening social nights playing "pub games" or taking part in panel games. Other activities included, inevitably, bingo, visits to local places of interest, stamp collecting and dancing to a record player donated by the League of Friends. These "extracurricular" activities were simply accepted by hospital staff as "part of the job". The Head Injuries Club would, as we shall see, become one of the precursors of today's charity, Headway. In an early example of multidisciplinary support, social workers attended the club regularly to offer support and advice. At the time the Club's work was pioneering and would lead to increased recognition of the needs of the head-injured at national and eventually international level. As part of this drive to promote the needs of the head-injured, Thackeray became a recognised lecturer at international conferences and a familiar face on television. Despite this, nationally progress was slow; even in 1982, 20 years after the club was founded, there were only two clubs specifically for victims of traumatic brain damage – one at the BAH and one in Nottingham; today, fortunately, there are many more.

Despite the success of the Head Injuries Club, it soon became clear that its members needed something more. They needed paid employment both as a source of

7. The Head Injuries Club

financial support and as a means of promoting self-respect. In 1964 The Head Injuries Rehabilitation Trust was formed. Thanks to the generous help of the Nuffield Provincial Hospitals Trust, the workshop was opened by the Bishop of Birmingham on 25th September 1967, although it had already been in operation a number of months by the time of its official opening. By June 1967 11 patients were working there, and numbers continued to increase as the value of the unit was recognised. The men attending (they all seem to have been men in the early days) attended each day and did industrial work which was constructive and interesting. Every patient was encouraged to develop their personality and abilities and the workshop was intended to provide these men with somewhere they could do useful work under expert supervision.

From the start, the main aim of the workshop was to allow patients with head injuries to make the transition back into the workplace with reducing levels of support, whilst accepting that some patients were too affected by their accidents to do so and would need lifelong sheltered support. Some of these problems were visible, others less so and the Accident Hospital was one of the first places where the mental health and personality changes, which commonly follow severe head injury, were first recognised and addressed. In line with the hospital's multidisciplinary approach, the head injury service included occupational therapists, clinicians, social workers, speech therapists, a social worker, a psychologist and a remedial gymnast. A maximum of 35 patients (males and females) between the ages of 16 and 65 years were accepted. Non-head-injured patients were also accepted if the service could be of benefit to them, but

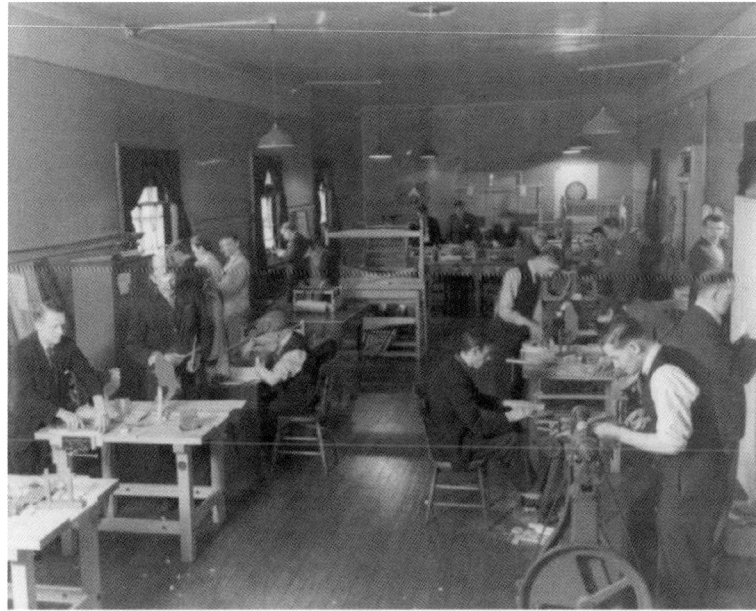

The sheltered workshop for patients with head injuries.

some patients with head injuries resulting in severe handicap or mental health problems could not be included. Each patient attended every day, but because the service was provided on an outpatient basis, the ability to attend depended to a degree on the availability of transport. The main emphasis of the Centre was on the establishment and maintenance of a good working routine. There were two large workshops where a variety of assembly, sorting and packing work was carried out. For example, rubber bath plugs were assembled and components for curtain rail fittings were counted, cut and packaged; cardboard boxes, box files and index cabinets were produced. Clerical work such as collating and stapling booklets and the making of birthday cards was undertaken. The Centre relied on firms for all the tasks it undertook, either to supply the work or purchase the end-products. It also had a woodwork area where patients made a variety of small items such as wine racks, small shelf units and mug trees; these items were offered for sale. At the same time as patients were reintroduced to the workplace, other aspects of rehabilitation were not forgotten and programmes of individually tailored development were carried out. These included the activities of daily living, re-education, social skills and overcoming speech and language problems. Charitable donations funded the creation of kitchen facilities used for patient education using the same approach as modern occupational therapists. Before discharge, each patient had to be capable of managing safely at home.

In general, individuals in the workshop started with simple assembly and packing tasks and then progressed to more complex machine work requiring a greater degree of manual dexterity and greater cognitive skills. Unusually for the time, support was offered by two discussion groups, one for patients, the other for relatives and friends.

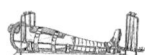

In 1979 Phillip Lockhart, supported by the Head Injuries Rehabilitation Trust, wrote to everyone in the country with an interest in the management of head-injured patients, a much more achievable task then, than it would be now. One of his first contacts was the equally determined Reg Talbott, principal social worker at Nottingham General Hospital. At the same time and entirely coincidentally, Sir Neville Butterworth placed an advert in a national newspaper seeking holiday accommodation for his brain-injured son and with Dinah and Barry Minton, also parents of a head-injured son, set out to find any support networks that already existed. Sir Neville was one of those contacted by Phillip Lockhart. These five individuals, carers and clinicians, called a meeting in October 1979 and Headway began, being registered as a charity the following year. Only 23 people attended that

7. The Head Injuries Club

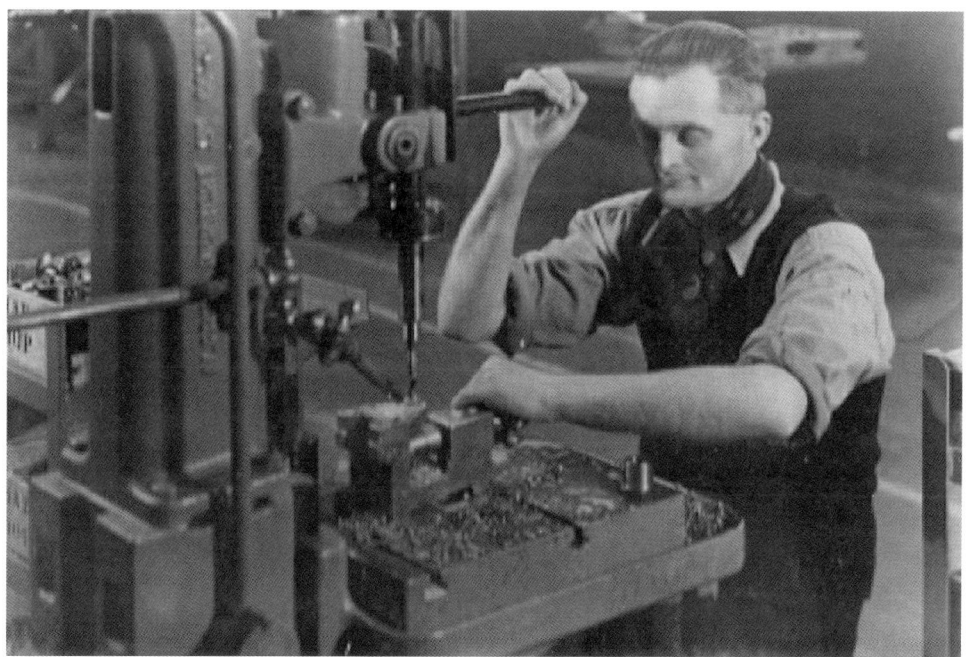

Returning to industrial work at the head injuries rehabilitation facility.

first meeting, a mixture of carers and clinicians, but by the time of the charity's first annual general meeting in 1981 there would be 22 local groups. The charity recognised that across the country the rehabilitation and support facilities for the head-injured had failed to keep pace with advances in treatment resulting in many more seriously impaired survivors; the first Headway House for long-term rehabilitation, respite care and hospital liaison opened in 1983 and others followed. Sadly, Phillip Lockhart did not live to see his dream of a national association for the head-injured become a reality.

It is worth pausing to review how the facilities for rehabilitation after trauma have changed in the years since the Accident Hospital closed. Accepting that the pioneering approach of the Accident Hospital in providing multidisciplinary support to those attempting to return to work represents a gold standard of care, how do today's seriously or critically injured fare?

The aim of trauma rehabilitation is to take a patient from point of injury, through surgical and medical management and return them to the highest possible levels of physical and psychological health, whilst integrating them back into society. As we shall see, many valuable lessons have been learnt as a result of the conflicts in Iraq and Afghanistan. Military rehabilitation, in which former Accident Hospital staff working at the Queen Elizabeth Hospital played a significant part, has been recognised as an example of rehabilitation service provision at its best. It is no coincidence that the distinguished chief of rehabilitation for the Armed Forces during and after the conflicts was a graduate of Birmingham Medical School. For the civilian population, provision is not so good. Indeed, it was clear that the NHS had neither the clinical capability nor capacity to manage the volume or complexity of the military casualties received in Birmingham.

Rehabilitation of trauma patients is complicated by multiple injuries, which cross organ and other traditional classification boundaries. These injuries affect the musculoskeletal and neurological systems as well as the skin, sensory organs and urogenital system. The NHS is organised to deliver rehabilitation based on single organ damage, such as brain injury, spinal cord injury or limb loss. Trauma patients frequently require therapeutic interventions from all these services simultaneously and therefore can rarely be managed effectively, or humanely, in the currently single-speciality focussed services of the NHS. Although every patient is required to have a "rehabilitation prescription", the integrated and coordinated services required to provide holistic care during return to maximal activity are simply, in many parts of the country, not there. It must also be said that where services do exist, the clinicians providing them are invariably working at full capacity and there simply isn't the space for every patient who needs support.

Psychological factors are a major influence on the long-term success of rehabilitation. Exposure to psychological trauma prior to injury, the death of colleagues, the near-death experience itself, disfigurement and perceived disability will complicate rehabilitation outcomes. Patients with similar injuries from similar circumstances may have widely different outcomes because of the individual's emotional response to the traumatic event. Similarly, even mild traumatic brain injury can have devastating consequences as it can impact on cognition and adaptability to life-changing events. However, these psychosocial factors are rarely pre-emptively addressed. In 2014-2015, there were approximately 994 occupied beds for all specialist rehabilitation in England. Around 20% of these beds were for trauma cases, giving a total of about 195 beds used for trauma patients in the whole of England. It has been estimated that only about 5% of cases treated in MTCs subsequently receive specialist rehabilitation. Figures suggest that each patient will stay for an average of approximately 75 days, therefore each bed will accommodate about five admissions per year; a total provision capacity of fewer than 1,000 admissions to specialist rehabilitation per year, for all NHS trauma patients in England. There are significant regional differences – provision ranges from one to eight beds for adult trauma patients per million population. Between half and two-thirds of the specialist rehabilitation units had insufficient staffing to manage a complex caseload. Involvement of rehabilitation medicine consultants within the major trauma centres varied, 18% of the major trauma centres had no rehabilitation medicine consultant input at all. Rehabilitation medicine support was particularly poor in London – with only one major trauma centre-funded session for a rehabilitation medicine consultant across the four networks in London.

The available NHS bed capacity is mainly targeted at managing patients with post-acute traumatic brain injury. These facilities do not have the capability or expertise to manage early trauma rehabilitation including multiple limb loss, complex musculoskeletal injury, spinal cord injury or burns and the multiple combinations of these injuries. The capacity of the NHS to expand and take on more trauma rehabilitation cases is negligible were such a requirement to arise from a major disaster or a terrorist event.

If rehabilitation is to be expanded then clearly it needs better funding, principally because it is seen as another drain on resources when other acute service requirements appear more pressing. They always will. The benefits of rehabilitation are realised financially by society as a whole – whilst the costs are met by the health service. The financial benefits are realised in reduced welfare payments, increased tax revenue, reduced social disruption through enhanced education opportunities, reduced criminality (brain injury) and reduced social care costs. The NHS simply doesn't feel it reaps the benefits of its rehabilitation efforts, although it is well established that there is a reduced demand on healthcare resources after appropriate rehabilitation.

Recent data suggests that only approximately 36% of patients had returned to their same employment six months after their injuries. Assuming there are 20,000 major trauma cases per annum and a national average salary for each patient, the average salary loss is £176.5m during that period (£353m pa), which is a loss in tax revenue of £31.2m (£64.4m pa). Benefit costs are difficult to quantify but a conservative estimate of loss to the exchequer for trauma every six months would be £58.2m. This does not consider other hidden costs such as the lost revenue from carers and spouses and takes no account of the human and other societal costs. England and Wales probably pay out about £40bn in health-related benefits per year. A small reallocation of resources to an effective rehabilitation programme would save money and lives and enhance the health of the nation.

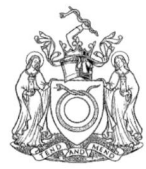

Fourth Interlude

War and Peace

EVERY YEAR THE solemnity of remembrance of those who died in the great conflicts of the twentieth century and smaller but no less lethal wars since feature the immaculate cemeteries of the Commonwealth War Graves Commission. Every single person who laid down their life is commemorated by a grave or by a name on a memorial. Yet this individual remembrance is, even today, a phenomenon little more than a century old. The first widespread establishment of British memorials followed the Boer War, the first examples of memorials appear to have followed the Crimean War in the middle of the nineteenth century. Before that, those who perished in battle or died of disease on campaign were quickly buried and forgotten. There are no mass graves on the battlefield of Waterloo. Although 50,000 people became casualties, only a handful of bodies have ever been found. Surprisingly to modern sensibilities, the bones of many of those who died on 18th June 1815 were ground up for fertiliser, much of which was purchased for use in the industrialisation of Britain's agriculture or for use in the refining of sugar. Making further use of a readily available resource, teeth extracted from the dead were combined into sets of "Waterloo teeth" and graced the dinner parties of Europe's wealthy. One assumes that many of those killed ridding Europe of a French megalomaniac failed to live long enough to develop significant dental disease, although it is not entirely clear how many corpses were needed to provide a full set of presentable teeth. It seems surprising therefore that at the same time as the bodies of the dead were being treated with such scant respect, the bodies of the living injured were the subject of genuine strides in the care of the wounded.

Fourth Interlude

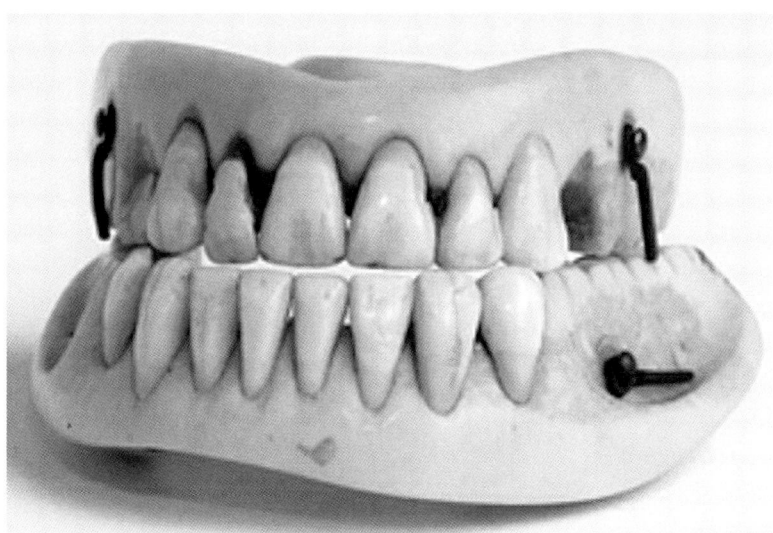

Waterloo teeth.

During the Napoleonic War, the great French surgeon Dominique Larrey developed both the battlefield ambulance and the concept of triage, the process by which the order of treatment for individuals is decided based on the severity of their injuries. At the same time, on the other side of the front line, Sir James McGrigor was laying the foundations of an organised army medical service, introducing field hospitals and improving standards of hygiene and cleanliness for patients and staff alike. It is a recurring facet of military medical history that many of his innovations were forgotten in a haze of complacency and ignorance by the time Britain became involved in its next major war in the Crimea.

The medical heroine of the Crimean War was, of course, Florence Nightingale who not only revolutionised nursing and made it respectable but was also the first to apply statistics to medicine and was a major figure in the establishment of public health, much of it achieved after she took to her bed in middle age. Despite a lifetime of ill-health, Florence lived to the age of 90. She was born in 1820 and named after the city of her birth (as one of her biographers commented, she was fortunate not to be born in Leghorn). After nurse training in Germany, at that time almost unthinkable for an upper-class young English women, she took the post of superintendent at the Institute for the Care of Sick Gentlewomen in Upper Harley Street. In 1854 with 38 volunteers and 15 nuns, she set off for the Crimean War. Although troops were far more likely to die of disease than of wounds, under Nightingale's formidable control, mortality was dramatically reduced, in many cases as a result of the introduction of simple hygiene measures such as hand washing and providing a simple but nourishing ration. Ventilation and sewerage were also tackled, reducing the levels of typhus, typhoid cholera and dysentery. Like so many of the great medical reformers, Nightingale realised that advances were best made by improving logistics such as supplies and food and that minds were best changed by incontrovertible evidence. She gave evidence to a Royal Commission on Army Health and would have as dramatic an effect on peacetime deaths as on deaths in war. Her other achievements included establishing nurse training as a profession for ladies rather than an occupation for slatterns, revolutionising hospital design, writing the first primer for nurses, introducing trained nurses into workhouses and establishing medical statistics as a means of influencing policy; tutored in mathematics by her father, she was among the first to use pie charts to present data. In 1859, Florence became the first female member of the Royal Statistical Society. Little escaped her notice and, despite never visiting the subcontinent, she was instrumental in improving the health of the Army in India as well as the general population following her conclusive linkage between poor sanitation and infectious disease. More importantly perhaps than all of this was that she made the care of the sick and (most relevantly for our purposes) injured, respectable.

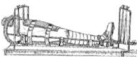

The war surgeon F.H. Albee commented of his experience in the First World War, *"There could only be one bright spot in this deplorable [situation] – that in the long run, humanity would benefit from the knowledge surgeons had gained in time of war."* We have already seen how the Second World War was a catalyst for the establishment of the Accident Hospital and we shall see, as the end of the story of the BAH approaches, how the conflicts in Iraq and Afghanistan ushered in the greatest advances in trauma care in modern times; advances in which Birmingham played a major part.

The Great War 1914-1918 was, as Albee remarked, also a pivotal moment in the development of care for the injured and in the recognition of orthopaedics as a speciality in its own right. As we have seen, Sir Robert Jones volunteered as a Territorial Army surgeon on the outbreak of war. Observing the poor quality of care of those injured in battle, and agitating for better treatment, he ended the War as Inspector of Military Orthopaedics and a major general with responsibility for more than 30,000 beds. Without doubt, Jones' single most important innovation was the introduction into conventional practice of his uncle's splint. Still an essential piece of medical equipment and present in every hospital's accident and emergency department, the Thomas splint transformed the management of femoral fractures and the chances of survival of those who sustained this injury.

Fourth Interlude

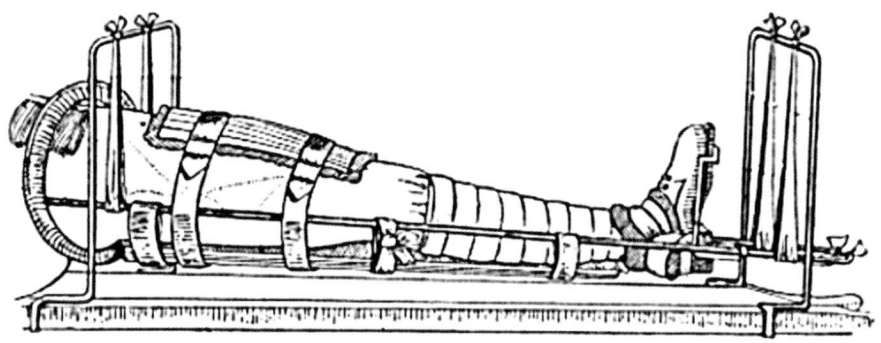

The Thomas splint.

The Thomas splint consists of an elongated metal U shape, the inner arm which is shorter, fitting against the inside of the patient's leg. The tops of the two arms are connected by a semi-circular padded collar sitting in the patient's groin. Straps suspended between the two arms support the patient's leg from below. Traction could be applied to the patient's leg by means of a tie, and a walking shoe could be fitted below the frame. Jones commented that his splint, which was cheap to manufacture and simple *"will enable any surgeon to treat his cases at home, with no more mechanical assistance than can be rendered by the village blacksmith and saddler, and the poorer class of sufferers will, at a small cost, be assisted as effectually as the wealthier classes"*. Jones' introduction of his uncle's splint would contribute significantly to reducing the mortality of battle related femoral fractures from its pre-war rate of 80% to around 15%. It also made transport of these patients much more comfortable. Other improvements associated with the medical services in the Great War included a deeper understanding of the management of blood loss, improved operative techniques for trauma victims and a mastery of the provision of medical care on the battlefield for hitherto unimagined numbers of casualties.

During World War II Thomas' splint would be combined with plaster of Paris to form the Tobruk splint. The Thomas splint has had an assured place in the management of femoral fractures, whether in war or civilian practice, ever since and learning to apply one correctly is a core skill for emergency physicians and orthopaedic surgeons alike. A statue of Sir Robert was unveiled at the opening of the Defence and National Rehabilitation Centre by the Duke of Cambridge in 2018 and the Robert Jones and Agnes Hunt Orthopaedic Hospital in Oswestry bears his name.

Orthopaedics and the care of the trauma victim were not only developing in Great Britain. We have already heard of Lorenz Bohler who taught William Gissane and whose Berlin unit was visited by Dr Matthew Burn before the Accident Hospital was founded. Bohler was a pioneer of accident surgery and had founded the AUVA Hospital in Vienna, which was a leading centre for fracture management. Bohler built his principles of treatment on those of Owen Thomas and Robert Jones, especially the importance of rest and rehabilitation.

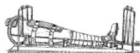

By the beginning of the Second World War, orthopaedics had been transformed from a speciality which concentrated on the treatment of deformities, often caused by tuberculosis, and treated with splintage, to a surgical speciality capable of addressing, at least in part, the injuries of modern warfare. Florey's work on antibiotics during the second world conflict had transformed the care of the injured so that patients with grossly contaminated wounds, who would certainly have died in earlier conflicts, had at least a chance of survival. Infectious diseases, in one form or another the curse of soldiers for generations, could be controlled. Effective blood transfusion became a practical aspiration following battlefield injury and the distinguished scientist Professor Solly Zuckerman (later Lord Zuckerman) carried out a series of classic experiments which at last clarified the true effects of blast on the bodies of the injured. Zuckerman was, for many years after the War, professor of anatomy at Birmingham Medical School, his *New System of Anatomy* was the guide to many generations of students during their time in the dissecting room.

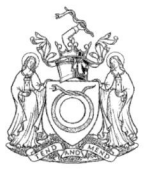

Chapter 8

Closure

AS THE TWENTIETH century drew towards its close, the writing was clearly on the wall for many of the small specialist hospitals which had provided the backbone of the health service. It was accepted that access to other specialties was required for the optimisation of patient care, although in some cases the tidying zeal of the growing cadre of administrators was probably as important a motivation. As so often with administrative logic, this resulted in closures which were neither sensible or necessary. It is a feature of administrative reorganisations which look logical on paper, that what is often lost is the intangible, the immeasurable, the soul of the institution. Loyalty and that willingness to go the extra mile are features of smaller bodies characterised by a caring approach to staff and patients alike, not to a process-obsessed medical mega-city. Only in recent years has the logic of an inevitable move towards huge hospitals been challenged.

Birmingham alone lost specialist hospitals dealing with skin diseases, brain surgery and neurological diseases, eye diseases, ENT and maternity services. It was therefore almost inevitable that the Accident Hospital would, in due course, follow suit. The lingering feeling remains that, administrative efficiency aside and clinical safety notwithstanding (the latter a useful shroud to wave to justify closures to be carried out for other reasons), something of the heart of the old NHS died with these smaller and now largely forgotten centres. In general, it might be accepted that larger hospitals offer the potential for better care than isolated specialist ones, but such decisions are best made on individual cases rather than following the political zeitgeist and there is little if any evidence to suggest that traumatised patients gained more from the subsequent closure and incorporation into a larger site than they lost in terms of clarity of clinical purpose and speciality integration.

In 1964 agreement was reached between the regional hospital board and the board of governors of the United Hospitals, that a new Birmingham Accident Hospital should be built on the Queen Elizabeth Hospital Centre site in Edgbaston as part of a series of developments taking place there. Two million pounds were set aside for the purpose of building a brand new 165 bed specialist trauma hospital. Ironically, the remaining staff of the BAH would eventually move to a new hospital on the Edgbaston site, but only in 2010.

A special committee was formed to develop the necessary proposals, attempting to ensure that the lessons of decades of specialist trauma practice would not be lost. It was agreed that the contractor should start work on the site in October 1970, completing the first phase of the building in 1972 and the second phase in 1974. It was hoped that the new hospital, although physically joined to other hospitals on the site and with much stronger links to the nearby University, would continue to possess an identity of its own. Just when it looked like a new day for the BAH and for the care of the injured was about to dawn, the plans were scrapped by the health minister Barbara Castle due to an economic crisis. Had this project been carried through to completion, it would have been the first modern major trauma centre in the UK by a matter of 30 years and would, even today, have been the country's only new-build specialist trauma centre.

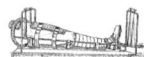

The Birmingham Accident Hospital closed its doors in July 1993 after 62 years of pioneering work in the management of severely traumatised patients. The closure of a freestanding trauma hospital was easier to justify with the perceived need for access to an increasing range of specialties in order to offer the best possible care. The hospital's own poet laureate, Edward Lowberry, was compelled to put pen to paper:

8. Closure

The Acci Is Dead: Long Live The Acci
(On the impending closure of the Birmingham Accident Hospital)

"Ask for the old Queen's," my neighbour said,
As I queued for a bus, bound for my new job
At the Accident Hospital. The Queen's was dead,
But a phoenix had sprung from its ashes. A quiet mob

Of patients crammed the entrance when I arrived:
So old a building for such a pioneer!
Was it a phoenix? or had the old one survived?
Our masters beamed, saying, "be of good cheer;

Your hospital will be transformed quite soon
With a new building, spacious and up-to-date!"
When visitors scanned my lab, that was the tune
I played, to calm their puzzlement. – Then fate

Struck, with its edict from the powers above:
"Forget your pipe dream, ditch the dolls' house,
That model hospital you've begun to love:
We can't afford to be so magnanimous."

From that bleak day I changed my tune, and when
Visitors came, I said "Just look around:
This lab was once a pre-Listerian
Surgical theatre; you're on historic ground!"

But visitors from every continent
Still came and went on coming, – not to see
A work of art, an ancient monument,
But for an update on our mystery.

50 years after the "Old Queen's" died
The phoenix which moved in, this pioneer,
Our much-loved Acci, now must step aside,
But it lives on, and will for many a year.

The "Acci"

Of all Birmingham's specialist hospitals, the Accident Hospital was the one in which the people of the city had invested the most, both financially and in terms of deep emotional commitment.

After its closure, many of the BAHs staff transferred to the Birmingham General Hospital before moving once again, in 1998, to Selly Oak Hospital. Neither bolt hole seemed likely to offer a long-term home. Its specialists had pioneered step changes in the reception, resuscitation, surgery and rehabilitation of the trauma victim and the same determination to provide optimum care for the injured would follow its former staff wherever they went. At the time it closed the BAH was recognised as the country's leading trauma centre: what was lost was a sense of community, a sense of separateness and of unity of purpose. Nevertheless, there were sufficient numbers of former Bath Row staff to keep alive some sense of the BAH's specific mission and this would survive, albeit less brightly, through the moves that followed until a final home was established at the Queen Elizabeth Hospital.

Critically injured patients continued to be taken straight to a major injuries unit, the medical staff continued to be organised into teams (four now rather than three) and care continued to be directed by a consultant. There were, of course, advantages to inclusion in a larger hospital and the most important of these was undoubtedly the opportunity to integrate with and work alongside other medical specialties and departments which had only been available on a peripatetic basis at the old hospital. Plans to separate the management of injured children and move them to the Birmingham Children's Hospital were dropped, although this move would eventually take place.

Ironically, the new Queen Elizabeth Hospital would be built on the site where, many years before, the foundation stone of a new Accident Hospital had been laid before the plan was abandoned.

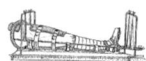

Eventually, in 2010, Selly Oak Hospital too would close and the remaining staff of the Accident Hospital would be transferred to the new Queen Elizabeth Hospital. By that time, in a dizzying sequence of changes, The Children's Hospital had been sold, the General Hospital had become the Children's Hospital and Selly Oak Hospital was in the process of demolition (since completed, save for its water tower).

At the Queen Elizabeth Hospital, as we shall see, under the leadership of Keith Porter (later Sir Keith Porter), world-class trauma care would flourish once more in response to the wars in Iraq and Afghanistan. Whilst the trauma capability was still based at Selly Oak Hospital, the UK Ministry of Defence made the decision to establish the Centre for Defence Medicine in Birmingham. In due course this would

8. Closure

become the Royal Centre for Defence Medicine and although it was unforeseen at the time, within a few months, injured service personnel would begin to arrive first at Selly Oak and then at the QEH. As a result, Birmingham's trauma service would be transformed and once again the city would be at the heart of innovation in trauma care.

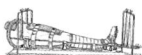

There were, inevitably, multiple reasons for closing the Accident Hospital. The hospital's parent health authority was insolvent and maintaining a single speciality hospital was becoming increasingly difficult. Access to the many specialties needed for the best possible care of the injured was no longer feasible on the Accident Hospital site. Saving the BAH might also have been more likely if it hadn't been the only one of its kind: scrapping a model which had been widely adopted might have been more difficult politically. The Birmingham-wide health services were also, as we have seen, undergoing a reconfiguration of services into which the BAH was swept. Fortunately, some of the important features of the old ways of working survived the transfers. The reputation of the old hospital meant that the injured were still brought to the former BAH clinicians and the team-based system continued, until it was swallowed up by changes in training and European working time directives. In true manager speak the new facility was renamed the South Birmingham Trauma Unit. The Major Injuries Unit still received direct transfers which were met by the trauma team. Within a short period the unit was handling a workload not dissimilar to its final year on Bath Row. By the time of the move to Selly Oak, on average, the new facility was seeing somewhere in the region of 50,000 new casualty cases each year. A similar number of physiotherapy appointments were carried out. A quarter of the trauma beds continued to be occupied by burns patients. The Infection Control Research Laboratory, which was also moved to a new location, survives to this day, the inheritor of the pioneering efforts of generations of Accident Hospital staff to reduce the impact of infection in the injured.

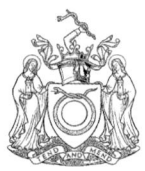

Chapter 9

A Hospital at War Again

PROF KEITH PORTER qualified at St Thomas' Medical School in 1974 with an established passion for the care of the injured. By the time he entered medical school he was aware of the reputation of the BAH and was determined one day to work there. The last consultant surgeon to be appointed to the BAH, in 1986, Keith Porter was, as we have seen, a pioneer of pre-hospital care, and more importantly for our story, it fell to him to keep the ethos of the hospital alive during its exile in Selly Oak Hospital and in its final home at the Queen Elizabeth Hospital. What could not have been predicted by the team of BAH clinicians who finally settled into the QEH in 2010 was that once again war and the care of its victims would dominate the history of trauma care in Birmingham into the twenty-first century.

The Centre for Defence Medicine was opened by the Princess Royal in 2001 and was granted the title "Royal" the following year. Its existence was the result of a report by Vice Admiral (then Captain) Sir Timothy Lawrence, the Princess Royal's husband. The centre was designed to be both a clinical and academic hub for the medical services of the Army, Royal Navy and Royal Air Force. Thus, by a combination of good luck (more) and good judgement (less) the ingredients of a centre for excellence in trauma management and the desire for a centre of military medical excellence were brought together and catalysed by the wars in Iraq and Afghanistan.

The Royal Centre for Defence Medicine was inevitably designated as the receiving hospital for all service personnel injured overseas, including those injured on active service. What nobody, least of all the politicians, had imagined was quite how

9. A Hospital at War Again

soon it would be that patients started to arrive and that what began as a trickle of the war-wounded would relatively rapidly become a flood. Whilst the trauma service was not ready to manage injuries on this scale, what it did have was a system, a model, that was based on the accumulated experience of the Birmingham Accident Hospital and which would serve as a prototype and foundation for all that followed. Alongside the military workload, the Queen Elizabeth's trauma teams would continue to develop a service for the people of the West Midlands, with survival becoming possible from levels of injury previously associated only with death. To function at this capacity, the hospital provided intensive care, laboratories, rehabilitation and social support and a full range of medical specialists. During the day there was a dedicated major trauma theatre, as well as two orthopaedic emergency theatres, a plastic surgery emergency theatre and two emergency hand surgery operating theatres. In addition, general surgical, neurosurgical and cardiothoracic theatres (and their staff) were also available if needed. At night, one theatre was always available and staffed and others could be opened as needed. The Major Injuries Unit had four beds with a combined intensive care and shock room capable of accommodating 11 and a remarkable 66 intensive care beds across the hospital. Consultants were required to live within 30 minutes of the hospital. At the time of the transfer of Accident Hospital staff from Selly Oak to the Queen Elizabeth Hospital, no-one could have predicted quite how soon and how rigorously these shiny new facilities would be tested.

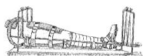

British troops entered Iraq as part of a coalition led by the United States of America on 20th March 2003, commencing what has been described as *"the most contentious war that the United Kingdom has ever fought"*. The decision to invade was justified by the now discredited "dodgy dossier" alleging the possession of weapons of mass destruction by the regime led by Saddam Hussein and the attempts of "hawks" in the US government to create a rationale for invasion based unconvincingly on the 9/11 attacks on New York. The intended collapse of the Iraqi regime was unsurprisingly rapidly achieved in the face of overwhelming coordinated force. Unfortunately, little attention was paid to what would happen afterwards and both UK and US forces found themselves trapped in a prolonged attritional campaign against shifting militias which would only end six years later. The situation was further irretrievably worsened by the decision to completely disband (but not disarm) the Iraqi security forces. A tin-ear to the sensitivities of the Iraqis and other Muslim nations characterised the US public political face before, during and after the war-fighting. As far as the UK was concerned, the predicament in which the military found itself was exacerbated by insufficient troop numbers, inadequate equipment and a failure of political and military leadership in forming a consistent concept of operations. In the early years of the War, the unprotected "snatch Land Rover" became something of a symbol of organisational failures. Significant numbers of casualties were inevitable. Perhaps uniquely in terms of conflicts involving the British Armed Forces, there was an immense wave of support for serving personnel against, at best, lukewarm support for the conflict itself.

The Western democracies had had a legitimate interest in Afghanistan since 9/11 as the operational base for the Islamic terrorists responsible led by Osama bin Laden. A number of operations followed which pushed the Taliban from power and into their tribal heartlands. In 2003, at the request of the newly established government of Afghanistan, NATO troops returned to the country as part of an International Security Assistance Force (ISAF) in an attempt to counter the growing Islamic extremist insurgency. At its height eight years later, this force would number more than 132,000 troops from 51 different countries. The campaign, which was handicapped once again by the lack of a consistent political and military strategy, would last until 2014 when the majority of British personnel left and the field hospital at Camp Bastion was closed. By that time, more than 450 personnel had lost their lives in addition to the almost 180 killed in Iraq.

From a medical point of view, the conflicts in Iraq and Afghanistan were transformational, not just for the Armed Forces Medical Services, but, as we shall see, for those responsible for receiving, treating and rehabilitating service personnel after their return to the United Kingdom. Pivotal to this response was the nucleus of staff imbued with the ethos and spirit of the Birmingham Accident Hospital.

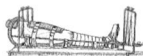

Service personnel in a conflict zone suffer injuries from many causes including sport, falling off, onto and under things, not to mention road traffic accidents and the occasional daftness of vigorous young men (and women) seeking to expend pent up energy in a stressful environment. More importantly, they also suffer the war wounds which are very often characteristic of the particular conflict in which they find themselves engaged. As the two campaigns became established, it rapidly became apparent that the "signature" injuries with which medical services, both on deployment and in the United Kingdom would have to contend were those caused by improvised explosive devices (IEDs). Although injuries as a result of gunfire were seen, more common were those resulting from standing on, or triggering, an IED, the resulting damage occurring in a pattern of which the medical services had no real experience.

9. A Hospital at War Again

Traumatic amputation of one or both legs was often accompanied by devastating injuries to the pelvis and external genitalia, although the frequency of the latter would in due course be reduced by rapid developments in body armour, resulting from a collaboration between Ministry of Defence technical experts and clinicians at the Royal Centre for Defence Medicine, examining clinical wound data. Triple amputees would in due course occur and, as methods of treatment improved, survive.

As the conflict in Afghanistan developed, so too did the treatment in theatre of injured personnel. Specific immediately life-saving techniques were taught to every soldier and a high proportion of combat troops were given extra medical skills and equipment; the skills of the unsung heroes of the conflict, combat medical technicians, were available in many cases immediately after wounding. The Medical Emergency Response Team carried on a Chinook helicopter brought consultant-led care to, or very close to, the point of wounding. At the field hospital in Camp Bastion casualties were received by a team led by an emergency medicine consultant and consisting of consultants from all the necessary specialties, guided for the first time by the deployment on operations of a CT scanner. Innovations, or not infrequently rediscoveries of established technologies, included giving blood and fluids via a needle into the bone marrow, tourniquets, agents designed to encourage blood clotting and prevent shock and new approaches to resuscitation with blood products. Every one of these innovations would in due course be accepted as standard in civilian practice. Because of the method of wounding, in general casualties occurred in small numbers at any one time. As a result, injured personnel could expect, and receive, world-class resuscitation and surgical intervention as soon as they reached the safety of the field hospital. Following this resuscitation and surgery, critically injured patients were then evacuated, usually within 24 to 48 hours, back to the UK by the Critical Care Air Support Team; effectively and actually a flying intensive care unit. They were received on arrival by the clinicians of the Queen Elizabeth Hospital Birmingham Trauma Unit consisting of both civilian and, increasingly as the conflict matured, military personnel led by Keith Porter and his team. Inevitably clinicians in Birmingham found themselves faced with casualties whose injuries were so severe that they would not have survived in any earlier conflict. Inevitably, this also brought its own particular challenges.

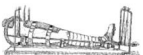

The challenge of dealing with wounds from war zones of a complexity and severity rarely seen before, and in quantities which could barely be imagined, led inevitably to the development of new techniques and the rapid refinement of established ones.

Surgical techniques developed remarkably quickly and clinicians developed a "feel" for the way particular injuries would behave. The fact that all injured personnel were evacuated to one hospital allowed for the relatively fast development of expertise by clinicians, which would not have been possible if the injured had been treated at multiple centres.

A good example of the refinement of an established method was the treatment of wounds with negative pressure, a technique initially pioneered at the BAH by the surgeon John Gower and found to be suitable for the complex wounds associated with improvised explosive devices.

The fact that the vast majority of the patients evacuated to Birmingham were young men (for obvious reasons, male patients were very much in the majority) at the peak of their physical fitness before injury, and now compromised by severe injuries brought its own challenges. As the BAH had very effectively demonstrated, the key to the best outcomes for trauma victims was multidisciplinary, multi-professional care led by experienced and expert clinicians. Inclusion of a wide range of professions allied to medicine as vital members of the team was, of course, second nature to those steeped in the Accident Hospital way of working.

Once the necessary life- and limb-saving surgery was complete, regaining mobility following amputation was obviously a major challenge, but other issues included maintaining morale within a military ethos, the psychological consequences of devastating trauma and the unforeseen need to address fertility after injuries to the external genitalia caused by improvised explosive devices. In due course developments in tissue sampling would allow a number of soldiers with such injuries to become fathers.

Crucial to the improvements in trauma care was new understanding of the effects of trauma on the body and the bodies response to it. This in turn led to a greater understanding of the best approaches to restoring normality to the critically injured body. The changes to patient treatment reflecting these new insights were implemented due to the combined efforts of clinicians, scientists and statisticians working together as they did at the BAH.

Injured service personnel returning to Birmingham would, as well as a wide range of medical clinicians including; anaesthetists, intensivists (intensive care specialists), general, plastic, chest and orthopaedic surgeons and rehabilitation consultants, be the beneficiaries of the efforts of physio- and occupational therapists, remedial instructors, psychologists, social workers, dieticians, prosthetists and podiatrists. All these individuals and more, including laboratory and technical staff, worked closely together as part of a multidisciplinary team; this was trauma care as Gissane and his pioneers wished so much to deliver it. The results were astonishing.

9. A Hospital at War Again

The rehabilitation of injured service personnel began in the Queen Elizabeth Hospital at the earliest opportunity, alongside complex general, orthopaedic plastic and other speciality interventions. The goal of returning patients to maximum function was in place before they left the intensive care unit. Throughout their journey to health, patients were discharged when safe and returned to the Queen Elizabeth Hospital or, as they continued to improve, to the Defence Medical Rehabilitation Centre at Headley Court in Surrey for further treatment or more intensive rehabilitation. Overall, on discharge from Headley Court, 95% of patients were independent in terms of the activities of daily living, 90% of amputees (around 50% of those with multiple limb loss) were able to walk independently over all terrains and 75% of triple amputees did not need a wheelchair for the activities of daily living. More than 90% of those who were unconscious when they first presented to medical care were also able to return to work. These results are the best monument not only to the complex and dedicated care the victims received and all those who delivered it, but equally to the sheer grit and determination of our injured service personnel. It can only be hoped that these clinical skills and commitment will be supported, funded and encouraged during years of relative peace ready for when they are needed again. Bitter experience suggests that this is unlikely, as they fall victim to spending constraints and the lack of moral courage amongst senior officers to defend them. Sadly also, as we have seen, this model of intensive multidisciplinary rehabilitation remains only an aspiration in many parts of the United Kingdom.

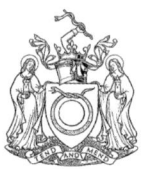

Afterword

DESPITE THE REPUTATION for excellence with which the Birmingham Accident Hospital came to be associated, and the recognition that specialist care saved lives and improved outcomes, the development of an effective service for the victims of trauma across the United Kingdom was shamefully slow. Whilst ready to recognise the BAH as a potential model for future services, such an approach was more widely reproduced in the USA than the UK. Clinicians in training went abroad, to the USA or South Africa, for experience of trauma care excellence. In truth, the BAH never spawned a single British unit in its own image. What it did do was to introduce into modern clinical practice not only a wide range of techniques designed to save the lives and improve the care of trauma victims, but it also demonstrated that the best trauma care required multidisciplinary teamwork, dedication and a profoundly serious approach.

Nevertheless, the drive for a coordinated clinical strategy for trauma continued, led very often by clinicians who had learnt their trade in Birmingham and were imbued with the "Acci spirit". Various reports commissioned by governments and academic bodies came and went, each with a title suggestive of profound disappointment at the lack of progress, each equally critical of the realities of individual patient care and the lack of an effective national strategy. Comparisons to national strategies for cancer, mental health or cardiac disease were made and forgotten, but little if anything changed.

Adding fuel to the debate was evidence from the USA, itself the beneficiary of developments pioneered at the BAH, that demonstrated that only 1% of deaths in specialist trauma centres were preventable whereas for smaller, non-specialist units, this figure was between 28 and 73%! The development of emergency medicine as a speciality in its own right, and the increasing availability of trained emergency medicine consultants, did lead to the establishment of increasing numbers of large emergency departments, but specialist trauma centres, with the exception of one or two internally generated units such as the Royal London, failed to be established. However, by 1988 the increasing evidence that poor care led to poor outcomes could no longer be ignored. A report that year by the Royal College of Surgeons found that one third of UK trauma deaths were potentially preventable. The report's authors also commented that effective care required training, multidisciplinary working, the concentration of trauma cases in specialist units and, equally importantly, effective and rapid pre-hospital medical intervention and transport. Unsurprisingly, the collection and analysis of patient data to inform and improve patient care was as lamentably poor as much of the patient care itself.

In 2007 an important report by the National Confidential Enquiry into Patient Outcomes, a statutory body established by Central Government, found that 60% of trauma patients received care that was, in their words, *"less than good practice"*. There were also striking differences between the survival rates at different hospitals. The following year, Lord Darzi, undersecretary of state for health announced that a national organised trauma system would be established across England and Wales; essential components of this new approach would be the recognition and establishment of regional major trauma centres in every region and effective pre-hospital arrangements for the immediate management and transfer of trauma victims. As a result of this new commitment, a series of working groups were established under the chairmanship of Prof Keith Willett (now Professor Sir Keith Willett) to address every component of an integrated trauma system from pre-hospital care to rehabilitation. Once again, a number of medical specialists with links to the BAH played significant roles.

Within three years it would be demonstrated that trauma systems saved between 450 and 600 lives each year. It would be estimated that by 2019 an 850 additional lives had been saved as a result of the newly established systems.

As a result, every area of England and Wales now has one or more dedicated major trauma centres capable of providing the necessary specialist surgery required by the victims of trauma and staffed by senior staff with extensive experience. Each patient's care is supervised and coordinated by a consultant and systems are in place to ensure that ambulances bypass smaller hospitals, bringing the seriously injured straight to the trauma centre without adding to clinical risks. Some trauma centres specialise in injured children, some only see traumatised adults, many do both, although major trauma in children is fortunately rare. As we have seen in the pioneering work of the Birmingham Accident Hospital, there are many components of a system designed to offer the best possible trauma care: as well as coordinated multidisciplinary management, these include research, education and data collection and are all part of the new system. At the same time, a new medical speciality of pre-hospital care has been established which means that the most seriously injured can be treated at the scene of their accident and that in many ways the resuscitation room and intensive care unit can go to them. The results achieved by the Medical Emergency Evacuation Team (MERT) in Afghanistan were in many ways crucial in establishing the value of such systems. The ubiquitous presence of charity-funded air ambulances means that patients can be transported rapidly and safely to the most suitable centre. Regional trauma desks at ambulance control ensure that the correct resources are allocated to each patient and that patients are received at the most appropriate facility.

The most critically injured, often those who have suffered major blood loss, chest injuries or who have suffered a cardiac arrest generate a "code red" call. This ensures that they are met on arrival by a team which includes a consultant trauma clinician, consultant anaesthetist, emergency medicine consultant and speciality consultants from, for example, neurosurgery or ophthalmology. A CT scanner and operating theatre are immediately available and a massive transfusion protocol ensures the immediate availability of blood and blood products. So many of these elements are part of the BAH's rich legacy to trauma victims and clinicians alike.

The Queen Elizabeth Hospital is the major trauma centre for Birmingham, the Black Country, Hereford and Worcester – one of three adult centres in West Midlands (the others being in Stoke and Coventry). The paediatric trauma centre is at Birmingham Children's Hospital. The CARE Team brings specialised care to the accident scene and the West Midlands Air Ambulance brings the patient to the trauma centre where they are met by a consultant-led team. In 2019 the Queen Elizabeth Hospital treated 652 patients with life-threatening or life-changing injuries.

In the 1950s William Gissane described his dream of a National Accident Service based around a small number of dedicated trauma centres. Finally, 70 years later, we have such a service. Gissane would have been pleased and proud, but perhaps would have raised a quizzical but polite eyebrow to find out that it took so long.

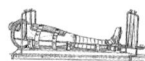

The Birmingham Accident Hospital has another legacy: in 1997 the charity Trauma Care was founded by Sir Keith Porter and two colleagues, one of whom had also worked at the BAH. For 25 years the charity has worked to promote multidisciplinary trauma care of the highest quality through education. Its coat of arms bears the Institute of Accident Surgery's motto "*Tend and Mend*" for these must be the twin guides of everyone charged with caring for the injured. If there were ever a clinical unit anywhere which embodied total dedication to the care of the injured with a pioneering spirit, a sense of social responsibility and an academic rigour, it was the Birmingham Accident Hospital of blessed memory and its achievements are something to which we should all aspire.

Further Reading

R. Jabet and J.P. Lucas. *A Concise History of Birmingham containing an account of its ancient state and the latest improvements.* Birmingham 1808.

James Drake. *Drakes' Picture of Birmingham.* Birmingham 1831.

Ian Greaves (Ed.) *Military Medicine in Iraq and Afghanistan: a comprehensive review.* CRC Press, London 2019.

The History of the Birmingham Medical School 1825-1925. A Special Number of the Birmingham Medical Review. Cornish Brothers Ltd., Birmingham 1925.

David Le Vay. *The Life of Hugh Owen Thomas.* E&S Livingstone Ltd., Edinburgh and London 1956.

P.M. Robinson and M.J. O'Meara. *The Thomas splint: Its Origins and Use in Trauma* Bone and Joint Journal Published Online:1 Apr 2009 https://doi.org/10.1302/0301-620X.91B4.21962.

Index

Index Note: locators in capitalised roman numerals refer to photograph gallery pages.

AA 88
Abraham, Edward 28
'ACCI' *see* Birmingham Accident Hospital
Accident Service Review Committee report 89
Adams Cowley, R. 70
Advanced Trauma Life Support 69-72
Afghanistan War 114-15, 120
air ambulances 76, 80, 120, VIII
airway constriction 70-1, 87, 90, 91-2
Albee, F.H. 104
Albert, Prince Consort *xxv*
Allan, F.G. 22
almoners 54-5, 96
Alpar, Mr Kaya Emin 92
ambulance fleet (late-1930s) 22
amputation and prosthetics *xvi-xvii*
anaesthesia 3-4, 20, 24, 44, 70, 72, 73
Andry, Nicholas 37
Anne, Princess Royal 112
antibiotics 28-9, 106
Ashley Miles, Professor 19, 28, VII
Ashley, Lady 28
Association of Industrial Medical Officers 12
Austin Motor Company 30, 33, 56-7, 64, 75, 88
Avery scales 33
Ayliffe, Professor Graham 92

bacteriology 28, 32, 33, 55, 61, 62, 74
Badger, Mr 59
Barnes, Stanley 12
Bath Row, Birmingham IV
Bedford Physical Training College 57
Bewes, Peter 92

Biggs, Ambrose, Mayor of Birmingham 8
Billington, William 11
Birmingham
  (18th and 19th centuries) *xviii-xxv*, 35, I
  (20th century) and Blitz 16-18, 82-6, 93
Birmingham Accident Hospital
  building and location V, VI, VIII
    building costs *xxiv*
  clinical staff and teams VII
    (1940s) 24, III
    at closure 93
    consultants *see* consultants
    juniors *see* junior doctors
    medical hierarchies (1940s) 44
    memories of *x*
    mobile medical response 79
    nursing staff and matron 24-5, 47
    registrars *see* registrars
    rota 53-4
    routine 46, 66-7
  closure and legacy 93, 107-8, 116-20, VIII
  departments
    casualty 58-60
    clinical photography 33
    dressing clinic V
    Hospital Infection Research Laboratory 92
    laboratory IV
    outpatients 21-2, 31, II
    pathology 55-6
    social services 30-1, 54-5, 96
  finances 11, 15, 22-3, 57, 93
    and funding 7, 28, 31, 33
    League of Friends 51, 96

Index

foundation *see* Birmingham Queen's Hospital
hospital magazine 48
Medical Society 50, 55
opening and early running 14-16, 20-3
    management board 15, 31
operating theatres 91, V
patient numbers 22-3, 56-7, 93
rehabilitation *see* rehabilitation
social club and Christmas festivities 47-50, III
Units
    Burns *see* Burns Unit
    Industrial Injuries 23-4, 32-3, 56, 65, 88
    Major Injuries 59-60, 91
    mobile surgical unit 74-8
    Road Injuries Research Group 64, 65, 88-9
    Wound Infection 28-9, 56
waiting room VI
wards *x*, 21, 47, 51, 87
    children's 63, VI
    wedding on II
Birmingham General Hospital *xxii-xxiii*, 12, 110
Birmingham Hospital Saturday Fund 5, 7
Birmingham Hospitals Contribution Association 33, 75
Birmingham Hospitals Council 12
Birmingham Medical School *xxii-xxv*, 44-5
Birmingham Post 83-4
Birmingham Pub Bombings 82-6
Birmingham Queen Elizabeth Hospital 12, 24, 46, 100, 108, 110, 112-13, 115-17, VIII
Birmingham Queen's Hospital 19, 21, 24, 51
    becomes 'The ACCI' *see* Birmingham Accident Hospital
    Charity Commission investigation 8-10
    early history *xxv*, 2-3, 11-13
        location and building I, II, IV
        and Queen's College *xxii, xxiv*, 1, 4, 6, 8-10

medical pioneers (19th century) 4-8
    during World War II 15-18
Birmingham Six 86
Birmingham Small Arms Company 23
Birmingham University *xxii*, 1, 11-12, 31, 45-6, 65, 92, 108
bleeding *xv-xvi*, 64, 66, 69, 71, 73-4
blood clots 56, 89
blood transfusion 88, 90-1
blood-letting 90
Bohler, Lorenze 15, 105-6
bone fractures and breaks 56, 71, 74, 89-90, 105
bone setters 37-8
brain and nerve function 71
Bramhope Tunnel Memorial 34
Brassey, Thomas 39-40
breathing 70, 71, 87, 90, 91-2
Breslau Jewish Hospital 26
Bright Eyes charity 93
British Orthopaedic Association 66
British Orthopaedic Society 41
Brunel, Isambard Kingdom 39
Bull, Dr John 19, 64, 65, 88
Bullivant, Miss E. (matron) 24
Burn, Dr Matthew 12, 106
Burns Unit 19, 23-4, 28, 29, 31-2, 50, 54, 61-2, 65, 89
Butterworth, Sir Neville 98

Cadbury's 33
Carson, Mr Hugh 22
casualty departments 57-8
Cater, Bill 91
Central Accident Resuscitation Emergency Team 79-80
Chain, Ernest 28
Chamberlain, Joseph 35
Champion, Professor Howard *xi*, 69-70
Charity Commission 8-10
children 63, 91-2, VI
cholera 1-2
Christmas festivities and social club 47-50

123

circulation 71
Clarke, Ruscoe 19, 53, 90-1, VII
Colebrook, Leonard 19, 23, 32-3, 61, 64, 65, III, VII
consultants 14, 20, 44-7, 49-50, 53, 57-60, 63, 66, 79, 80, 81, 93, 113
 see also personal names; surgeons
convalescent homes 7-8, 31, 55
Cox, Edward Townsend 2
Crimean War 103-4

Daniels, Sister 16
Darzi, Lord 119
Defence Medical Rehabilitation Centre 117
Diana, Princess of Wales 50, VIII
Dickson, Dr Graeme *xi*, 92-3
disinfection 61
Donovan, H. 22
Donovan, T.S. 22

Elizabeth II, Queen 33
emergency departments 57-8
Essex-Lopresti, Peter 24, VII
Etherington, Dr John *xi*

Farrell, Roger *xi*
First World War 11-12, 41, 104
Fleming, Sir Alexander 28
Florey, Dr Ethel 28, VII
Florey, Howard 28-9, 106
Foster, Balthazar Walter 4-5
Friends (Quakers') Ambulance Unit 25
funding for rehabilitation 101

Galloway, Sister 16
Gamgee, Sampson (Sam) 5-6, 7
General Electricity Company 23
George VI, King IV
Gissane, William 18-20, 22, 23, 25-7, 30, 50, 54, 57, 58, 62, 64, 75, 81, III, VII
GKN 33
Glasgow Coma score 71
Gower, John *xi*, 116

Greaves, Ian *x*
Guest, Keen and Nettlefold (GKN) 33
Guttman, Ludwig 26-7

Hall Edwards, Dr John 6, 41, II
Hannon, Sir Patrick 33
head injuries 94-101
Head Injuries Club 96-7
Head Injuries Rehabilitation Trust workshop 97-8
Headley Court 117
Headway charity 96, 98-9
Heating Appliances and Fireguards Act 1952 33
Hicks, J.H. 89-90
Horner, Maggie *xi*
housemen 44
Hunter, John 55
Hunterian Lecture 29
Hunterian Professorship 24, 29, 55
Huskisson, William *xviii*, 35
Hyden, Sister 16

ICI Metals 33
industrial health and safety 25-6, 33, 34-42, 62
 Industrial Injuries Unit 23-4, 32-3, 56, 65, 88
 Industrial Medicine and Burns Research Unit 64-5
infection control 28-9, 92
Institute of Accident Surgery 66
Institute of Orthopaedic Surgery 41
IRA 84, 86
Iraq War 113-14

Jackson, Douglas MacGilchrist 19, 29, VII
Jones, Dr J. Rhaiadr 23
Jones, Sir Robert 38, 40-2, 104
junior doctors 14, 43-7, 49-50, 57, 88

Kingsley, Charles 8, 21

Index

Larrey, Dominique 103
League of Friends 51, 96
Lind, Jenny 2-3
Lister, Joseph 4
Liston, Robert *xvii*, 3
Liverpool's Cripples' Champion 38
Llandudno convalescent homes 7-8
Lockhart, Phillip 96, 98-9
Lombard RAC Rally 80
London, Nick 76
London, Peter 75-6, 96, VII
Lowbury, Edward 19, 32, 53, 60-1, VII

Macmillan, Harold 86
Major Injuries Unit 59-60, 91
Manchester Ship Canal 40, 41
Matherson, Tom 76
McGrigor, Sir James 103
Medical Emergency Evacuation Team 120
Medical Research Council 19, 23-4, 28, 32-3, 56, 65, 88
Medical Society 50, 55
medical students *x, xxii,* 1-2, 44-7, 57
mental health 2, 97-8, 100
Mercedes dealership 80
Merck & Co *xv*
Midlands Air Ambulance 80
military medical history 103-6, 112-17
Millard, Peter *xi*
Minton, Dinah and Barry 98
mobile surgical unit 74-8
Mulberry explosion 82-3
Muller, Olga 29, VII

Napoleonic War 102-3
National Confidential Enquiry into Patient Outcomes 119
National Health Service 57, 91, 100-1
neurology 26-7
neurosurgery 57
Nightingale, Florence 103-4
Nottingham General Hospital 98

Nuffield Provincial Hospitals Trust 97
nurses 1, 24-5, 43, 104

operating theatres 91, V
orthopaedics 16, 37, 40-2, 66, 104-6
outpatients department 21-2, 31, 76, II
oxygen 72

paramedics 79-80
pathology department 55-6
Phillips, Lesley 16
physiology 4
physiotherapy 30, 57
Pirogov, Nikolay Ivanovich 3
Porter, Professor Sir Keith *ix, xi,* 75, 79, 80, 110, 112, 115, 120, VII
post-mortem examinations 56
pre-hospital care 75-81, 84-5
Princess Michael of Kent 50-1
Provisional Board of Management (1940) 16

Queen Elizabeth Hospital 12, 24, 46, 100, 108, 110, 112-13, 115-17, 120, VIII
Queen's College *xxii, xxiv,* 1, 4, 6, 8-10
Queen's Hospital *see* Birmingham Queen's Hospital

radiology (X-ray) 6, 41, 88
railways 39-40
registrars 22, 24, 44, 45, 53-4, 63, 76
rehabilitation 15, 23, 26-7, 33, 60, 61-2, 95-101, 105-6, 117
   Austin Motor Company 56-7
   convalescent homes 7-8, 31, 55
   funding 101
   social services 30-1, 54-5, 96
   Stanford Hall 42
   see also trauma care, principles of
Rehabilitation of Person's Injured by Accident (1939) 13, 14
religion *xxiv*
Road Injuries Research Group 64, 65, 88-9
Roberts, Barbara 64

Rook, Dr John R. 24
Rowley, Miss M.J. 22
Royal Centre for Defence Medicine 112-13
Royal Orthopaedic Hospital 16

Salt, Titus 36
Sands Cox, William *xix, xx-xxv*, 3, 4, 7, 8-11, 11
Savage, Miss 95
Scott Review (1972) 89
Second World War *see* World War II
Selly Oak Hospital 110-11, 112
senior house officers 44, 53
Sevitt, Dr Simon 19, 55-6, 88, 89
skin diseases 24, 28
Snow, John 1-2
social services department 30-1, 54-5, 96
sporting events 80
Squire, Professor John 23-4, 64-5
Stewart, Dr Donald 12, 64, 88
Stoke Mandeville 26-7
strike (December 1989) 79
Styner, James K. 69-72
surgeons
    early professional status *xx*, 3
    surgical practice 58-9, 62-3, 91-2
    see also consultants
Sutcliffe, Dr Anne *xi*

Talbott, Reg 98
teeth 102-3
Telford, Thomas 39
Temple Row, Birmingham *xx-xxi*
Thackeray, Jack 95-6, VII
Thomas, Colin 91
Thomas, Evan 37
Thomas, Hugh Owen 37-8, 40-1
    Thomas splint 41, 71, 78, 104-6
thromboses 56, 89
Topley, Betty 24
Tovey, Hatty *xi*
tracheostomy 87, 90
Trauma Care charity 120

trauma care, principles of
    20th century 14-15
        Advanced Trauma Life Support 69-70
    21st century 119-20
        liquids given and "golden hour" 90
    multidisciplinary approach 30, 116
    national bed capacity 100-1
    archaeological evidence *xiv-xvii*
    deaths and survivor effects *xiii-xiv*, 68-74, 101, 118-19
    see also rehabilitation
trepanning *xiv, xv*

United Birmingham Hospitals 20-1
United States of America 27, 41, 69-70, 118
University of Birmingham *xxii*, 1, 11-12, 31, 45-6, 65, 92, 108

Vernon, Sydney 13, 15
Victoria, Queen *xxv*, 3, 6
volunteers 50

W&T Avery 33
Walker, Michael *xi*
Walker, Thomas 40
Waller, Augustus Désiré 4
Waller, Augustus Volnay 4
war memorials 102
Ward, William Humble, 2nd Earl of Dudley 11
Warnfield, Samuel *xxiv*
West Midlands Ambulance Service 79
Williams, Dr R.E. 19, 28
Withering, William *xxiii*, 2, 4
Wolfson, Dr Joe 20
World War I 11-12, 41, 104
World War II 16-18, 20-3, 25, 27-8, 30-2, 53
Wright, Sir Almroth 32

X-ray (radiology) 6, 41, 88